The Unofficial Guide to Radiology

100 Practice Orthopaedic X-rays

SECOND EDITION

EDITION

2

The Unofficial Guide to Radiology

100 Practice Orthopaedic X-rays

Edited by

Christopher W. Gee MBChB, MSc, FRCSEd
(Tr&Orth), MFSTEd
Interim Clinical Director and Consultant Orthopaedic Surgeon
NHS Golden Jubilee
Glasgow, Scotland

Honorary Senior Clinical Lecturer, University of Glasgow
Scotland

Education Lead for the West of Scotland Orthopaedics Rotation

Series editor
Zeshan Qureshi BM, BSc (Hons), MSc, MRCPCH,
FAcadMEd, MRCPS (Glasg)
Paediatric Registrar
London Deanery
United Kingdom

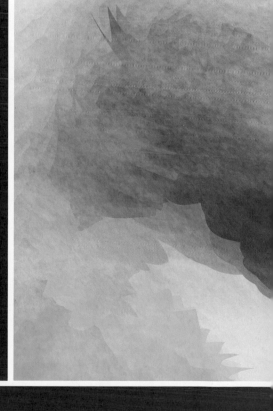

ELSEVIER

First edition 2019. Published by Zeshan Qureshi.

Notices

Practitioners and researchers must always rely on their own experience and knowledge in evaluating and using any information, methods, compounds or experiments described herein. Because of rapid advances in the medical sciences, in particular, independent verification of diagnoses and drug dosages should be made. To the fullest extent of the law, no responsibility is assumed by Elsevier, authors, editors or contributors for any injury and/or damage to persons or property as a matter of products liability, negligence or otherwise, or from any use or operation of any methods, products, instructions, or ideas contained in the material herein.

ISBN: 978-0-443-10919-5

Content Strategist: Trinity Hutton
Content Project Manager: Tapajyoti Chaudhuri
Design: Hitchen Miles
Marketing Manager: Deborah Watkins

Printed in India

Last digit is the print number: 9 8 7 6 5 4 3 2 1

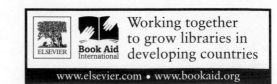

I would like to dedicate the second edition of this book to my wonderful and supportive wife of 15 years Gemma, my daughter Ivy who brightens every day and my 3 cats Mochi, Miss Moppet and Maisie.

I would also like to dedicate this book to all the patients currently on Orthopaedic waiting lists and hope that those who read and learn from this book one day have the same privilege I have every single day, treating people with orthopaedic problems, and seeing patients regain the function they require to live day to day.

Christopher Gee

Contents

Series Editor Foreword

The Unofficial Guide to Medicine is not just about helping students study, it is also about allowing those that learn to take back control of their own education. Since its inception, it has been driven by the voices of students, and through this, democratized the process of medical education, blurring the line between learners and teachers.

Medical education is an evolving process, and the latest iteration of our titles has been rewritten to bring them up to date with modern curriculums, after extensive deliberation and consultation. We have kept the series up to date, incorporating new guidelines and perspectives from a wide range of students, junior doctors and senior clinicians. There is greater consistency across the titles, more illustrations, and through these and other changes, I hope the books will now be even better study aids.

These books though are a process of continual improvement. By reading this book, I hope that you not only get through your exams but also consider contributing to a future edition. You may be a student now, but you are also the future of medical education.

I wish you all the best with your future career and any upcoming exams.

Zeshan Qureshi
November 2022

Introduction

Following history taking and examination, taking X-rays of the affected area is often an important part of the assessment of a patient with a suspected fracture or musculoskeletal condition.

When faced with X-rays of a bone or joint, it can be difficult knowing where to start looking for an abnormality and how to describe an abnormality, whether it be a fracture, dislocation, joint problem or bone lesion, and how to link this to the overall patient management. However, like most of medicine, the key is having a systematic approach and getting lots of practice!

The Unofficial Guide to Orthopaedic Radiology guides you through a series of 100 trauma and orthopaedic X-rays. The cases have been selected by orthopaedic surgeons and radiologists to cover common and important X-ray findings, and include common fractures, subtle abnormalities and less common lesions such as bone tumours.

The cases are structured to be as clinically relevant as possible and follow the highly successful approach used in The Unofficial Guide to Radiology. Each case includes a clinical history with relevant examination findings. The large, high-quality images offer you the chance to practise interpreting the X-rays as you would in real life. Turning the page reveals a systematic assessment of the X-rays, with clear, on-image annotations highlighting the pertinent findings. Technical information is followed by assessment of fractures, joints, soft tissue, background bone, bone lesions, a summary/differential and then investigations/ management. Note that while the management of these cases have been discussed, it is more important during medical school and early training to focus on being safe and making the diagnosis. If you are ever in doubt, do not be afraid to ask for help.

By practising our systematic approach, you will become confident in assessing, interpreting and presenting orthopaedic X-rays.

In this second edition, there are additional 300 bonus questions, which will allow you to learn more of the theory for each of the cases.

Additionally, we want you to get involved! This textbook has mainly been written by junior doctors and students just like you because we believe:

- That fresh graduates have a unique perspective on what works for students. We have tried to capture the insight of students and recent graduates to make the language we use to discuss complex material more digestible for students.

- That texts are in constant need of being updated. Every student has the potential to contribute to the education of others by innovative ways of thinking and learning. This book is an open collaboration with you.

Realistic clinical history

Case
13

A 76-year-old woman has been brought to hospital by her husband after she tripped down the stairs at home. She describes landing on her outstretched right hand. She is complaining of pain in the wrist and states that it looks abnormal. There is no significant past medical history. On examination, there is an obviously deformed forearm, with tenderness over the wrist. Distal pulses are present and motor and sensory function is preserved. The injury is closed.

AP and lateral X-rays of the right wrist are requested to assess for a fracture.

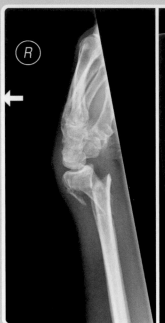
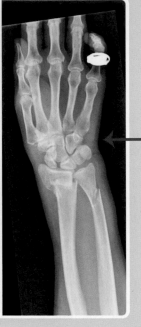

Large, high quality image to assess

REPORT – DISTAL RADIUS AND ULNAR FRACTURES

27

Detailed report following a standard format

TECHNICAL INFORMATION
Patient ID: Anonymous.
Area: Right wrist.
Projection: AP and lateral.
Technical adequacy:
- Adequate coverage.
- Adequate exposure.
- The patient is not rotated.

● FRACTURE DETAILS
There is a fracture involving the distal radius.
The fracture is transverse, comminuted and extraarticular.
There is marked dorsal (posterior) and mild radial (lateral) displacement along with dorsal (posterior) angulation.

There is shortening.
There is no rotation.
There is a fracture involving the distal ulna.
The fracture is oblique, simple and extraarticular with marked dorsal (posterior) angulation.
There is no translational displacement.
There is no rotation.
There is no shortening.

● JOINTS
There is no subluxation or dislocation.
There are no loose bodies.
There is no effusion or lipohaemarthrosis.
There are no arthritic changes.

● SOFT TISSUES
There is soft tissue swelling.
There is no surgical emphysema.

● BACKGROUND BONE
The background bone is normal.

● BONE LESIONS
There is no bone lesion present.

X-ray review areas specifically highlighted

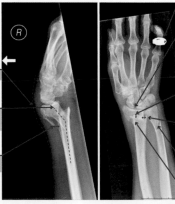

Clear annotations highlighting the major x-ray findings

Soft tissue swelling

Marked dorsal angulation of the ulnar fracture

Dorsal displacement of the radial fracture

This ring needs removal before the hand swells

Widening of the scapholunate interval raises the suspicion of a scapholunate ligament injury. This is the so called Terry Thomas or Madonna sign

Shortening of the radial fracture

Mild lateral displacement of the radial fracture

Oblique distal ulnar fracture

Transverse distal radial fracture

SUMMARY AND DIFFERENTIAL
Both X-rays demonstrate a dorsally angulated and displaced distal radial fracture with an associated distal ulna shaft fracture.

INVESTIGATIONS AND MANAGEMENT
Analgesia should be provided.

The fracture should undergo closed reduction in the ED under one of many suitable techniques including sedation, haematoma block or Biers block. A moulded back slab should be applied. Postreduction X-rays should be taken.
A referral should be made to orthopaedics who may consider surgical fixation.

Investigations and management plan put the x-ray in the context of the overall clinical management

Acknowledgements

Thank you to the following contributors for their contribution to the first edition:

Mark Rodrigues
Alexander Young

Abbreviations

AC	acromioclavicular	**IV**	intravenous
ACJ	acromioclavicular joint	**MRI scan**	magnetic resonance imaging scan
ACL	anterior cruciate ligament	**MT**	metatarsal
AP	anteroposterior	**MTP**	metatarsophalangeal
ASB	anatomical snuff box	**MUA**	manipulation under anaesthetic
ATLS	advanced trauma life support	**NSAIDs**	nonsteroidal antiinflammatory drugs
AVN	avascular necrosis		
CRIF	closed reduction internal fixation	**ORIF**	open reduction internal fixation
CRP	C-reactive protein	**PIPJ**	proximal interphalangeal joint
CRT	capillary refill time	**PR**	per rectum
CT scan	computed tomography scan	**RICE**	rest ice compression elevation
DIPJ	distal interphalangeal joint	**ROM**	range of movement
DISH	diffuse idiopathic skeletal hyperostosis	**RTC**	road traffic collision
		SI	sacroiliac
ED	emergency department	**SUFE**	slipped upper femoral epiphysis
FBC	full blood count	**TB**	tuberculosis
GP	general practitioner	**THR**	total hip replacement
ID	identification	**TIA**	transient ischaemic attack
IP	interphalangeal	**TLSO**	thoracolumbar sacral orthosis

Contributors

SERIES EDITOR

Zeshan Qureshi
BM, BSc (Hons), MSc, MRCPCH, FAcadMEd,
MRCPS (Glasg)
Paediatric Registrar, London Deanery,
United Kingdom

EDITOR

Christopher W. Gee
MBChB, MSc, FRCSEd (Tr&Orth), MFSTEd
Interim Clinical Director and Consultant
Orthopaedic Surgeon, NHS Golden Jubilee
Glasgow, Scotland

Honorary Senior Clinical Lecturer, University of
Glasgow, Scotland

Education Lead for the West of Scotland
Orthopaedics Rotation

HAND AND WRIST

A 37-year-old right-hand-dominant female office worker fell at a Christmas party, landing on her outstretched right hand. She is brought into the ED. There is no significant past medical history. On examination, there is no obvious swelling or deformity but tenderness is elicited on palpation of the anatomical snuffbox and with pulling of the thumb. Distal pulses are present and sensory and motor function is preserved. The injury is closed.

Scaphoid series X-rays of the right scaphoid are requested to assess for a fracture.

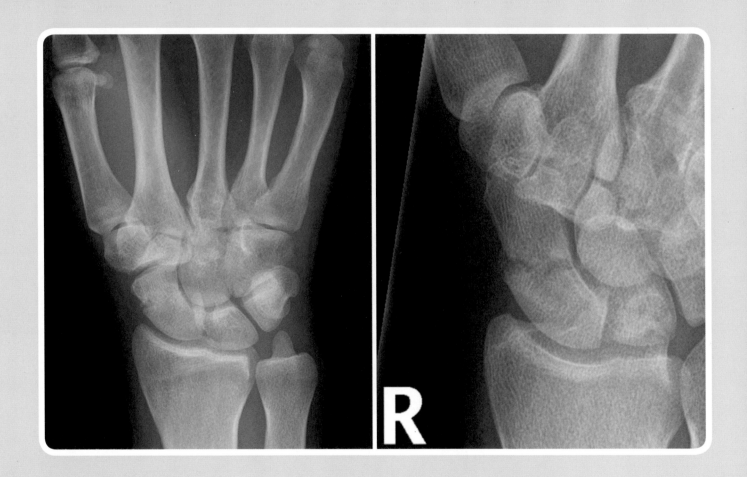

TECHNICAL INFORMATION

Patient ID: Anonymous.
Area: Right scaphoid.
Projection: AP and oblique.
Technical adequacy:

- Adequate coverage but additional views (lateral and angled AP) are required to complete the scaphoid series.
- Adequate exposure.
- The patient is not rotated.

● FRACTURE DETAILS

There is a fracture involving the midportion (waist) of the scaphoid.

The fracture is transverse, comminuted and extraarticular.

There is minimal displacement and comminution.

There is no angulation.

There is no rotation.

There is no shortening.

● JOINTS

There is no subluxation or dislocation.

There are no loose bodies.

There is no effusion or lipohaemarthrosis.

There are no arthritic changes.

● SOFT TISSUES

There is no soft tissue swelling.

There is no surgical emphysema.

● BACKGROUND BONE

The background bone is normal.

● BONE LESIONS

There is no bone lesion present.

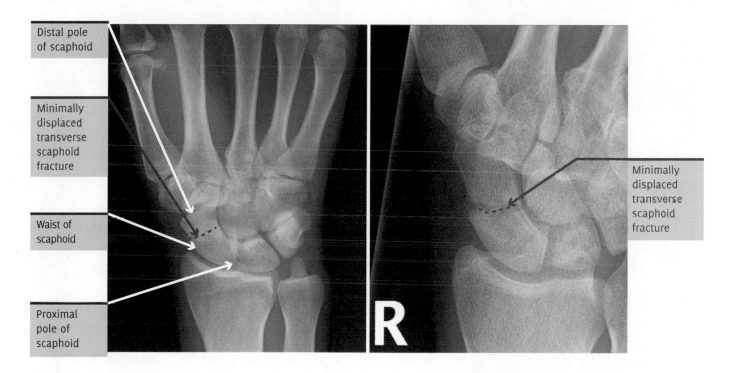

Distal pole of scaphoid

Minimally displaced transverse scaphoid fracture

Waist of scaphoid

Proximal pole of scaphoid

Minimally displaced transverse scaphoid fracture

R

SUMMARY AND DIFFERENTIAL

These X-rays demonstrate a minimally displaced scaphoid waist fracture.

INVESTIGATIONS AND MANAGEMENT

Appropriate analgesia should be provided.

The other views from the scaphoid series should be reviewed to assess for alignment of the carpal bones, in particular, the scapholunate and capitolunate angles. A below-elbow back slab should be applied, and referral made to fracture clinic. Whilst it is likely that this would be managed nonoperatively, operative management may be considered depending on the results of the full scaphoid X-ray series.

A 35-year-old right-hand-dominant woman fell over whilst skiing. She reports landing awkwardly on her left thumb. She presents to the ED. There is no significant past medical history. On examination, the patient has a swollen and tender left thumb. She is unable to move the thumb at the carpo-metacarpal joint because of pain. Distal pulses are present and sensory and motor function is preserved. The injury is closed.

AP and lateral X-rays of the left thumb are requested to assess for a fracture.

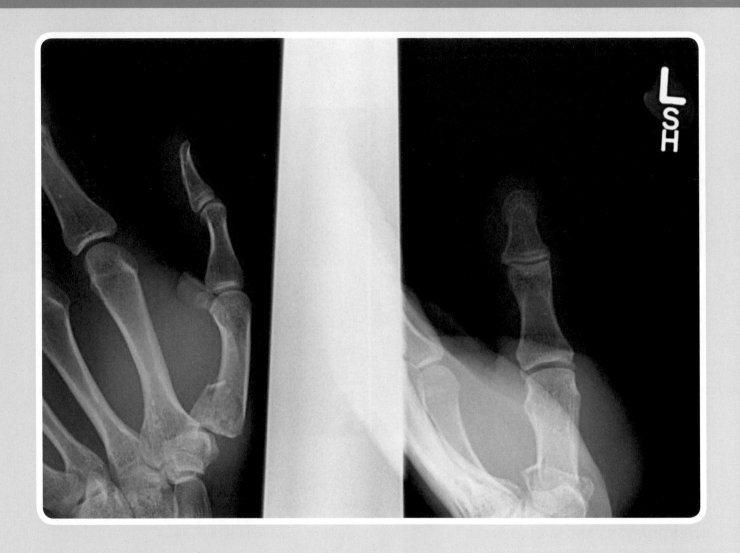

TECHNICAL INFORMATION

Patient ID: Anonymous.
Area: Left thumb.
Projection: AP and lateral.
Technical adequacy:

- Adequate coverage.
- Adequate exposure.
- The patient is not rotated.

● FRACTURE DETAILS

There is a fracture involving the proximal aspect of the first metacarpal.

The fracture is oblique, simple and juxta articular.

There is no displacement.

There is no angulation.

There is no rotation.

There is shortening (difficult to estimate) and impaction of the fracture fragments.

● JOINTS

There is no subluxation or dislocation, in particular, the first carpo-metacarpal joint remains congruent.

There are no loose bodies.

There is no effusion or lipohaemarthrosis.

There are no arthritic changes.

● SOFT TISSUES

There is no soft tissue swelling.

There is no surgical emphysema.

● BACKGROUND BONE

The background bone is normal.

● BONE LESIONS

There is no bone lesion present.

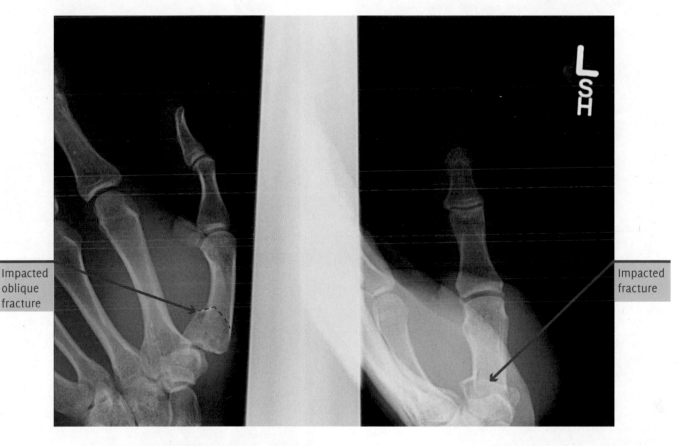

Impacted oblique fracture

Impacted fracture

SUMMARY AND DIFFERENTIAL

These X-rays demonstrate an impacted fracture at the base of the first metacarpal. This fracture may be intraarticular and is called a *Bennett's fracture*.

INVESTIGATIONS AND MANAGEMENT

Appropriate analgesia should be provided.

The patient should have a Bennett-type back slab applied and have repeat X-rays. A referral should be made to fracture clinic.

If repeat imaging confirms an intraarticular fracture with displacement, or this is a concern, then a CT scan should be requested to better assess the articular surface. Displaced, intraarticular fractures require MUA and K-wire fixation. If the fracture is extraarticular, then it can often be treated nonoperatively unless widely displaced.

Case

3

A 35-year-old right-hand-dominant female surgeon presents to the Minor Injuries Unit, having caught her left little finger making the bed. There is no significant past medical history. On examination, there is a haematoma over the dorsal aspect of the 5th DIPJ. She is unable to extend the finger. The finger is well perfused with intact sensation. She is unable to extend the DIPJ. The injury is closed.

AP and lateral X-rays of the left little finger are requested to assess for a fracture.

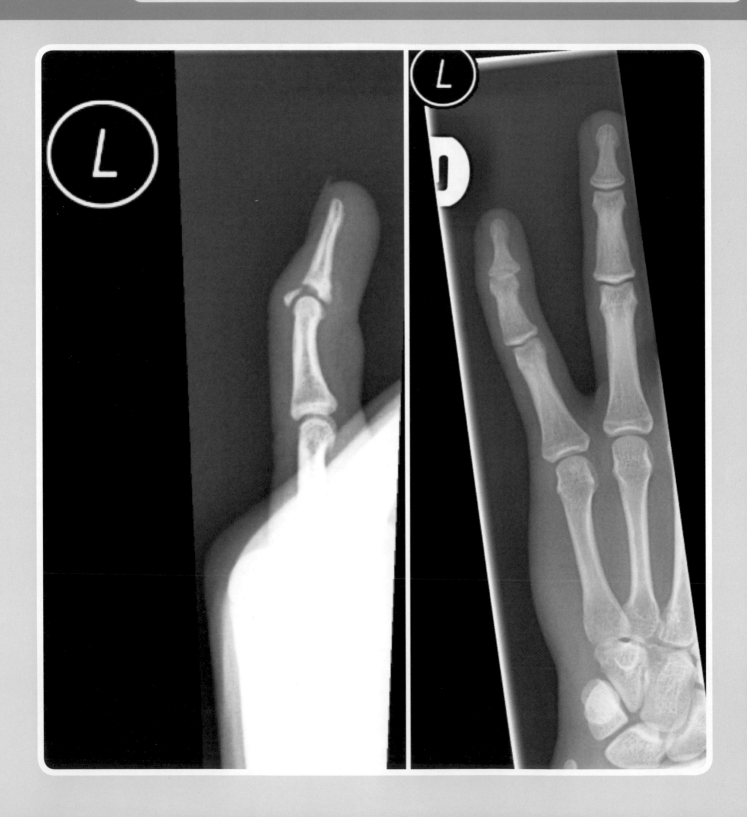

TECHNICAL INFORMATION

Patient ID: Anonymous.
Area: Left distal phalanx of the 5th finger.
Projection: AP and lateral.
Technical adequacy:

- Adequate coverage.
- Adequate exposure.
- The patient is not rotated.

FRACTURE DETAILS

There is an avulsion fracture involving the base of the distal phalanx of the little finger.

The fracture is triangular, simple and intraarticular.

There is minimal displacement.

There is no angulation.

There is no rotation.

There is no shortening.

JOINTS

There is no subluxation or dislocation of the DIPJ.

There are no loose bodies.

There is no effusion or lipohaemarthrosis.

There are no arthritic changes.

SOFT TISSUES

There is no soft tissue swelling.

There is no surgical emphysema.

BACKGROUND BONE

The background bone is normal.

BONE LESIONS

There is no bone lesion present.

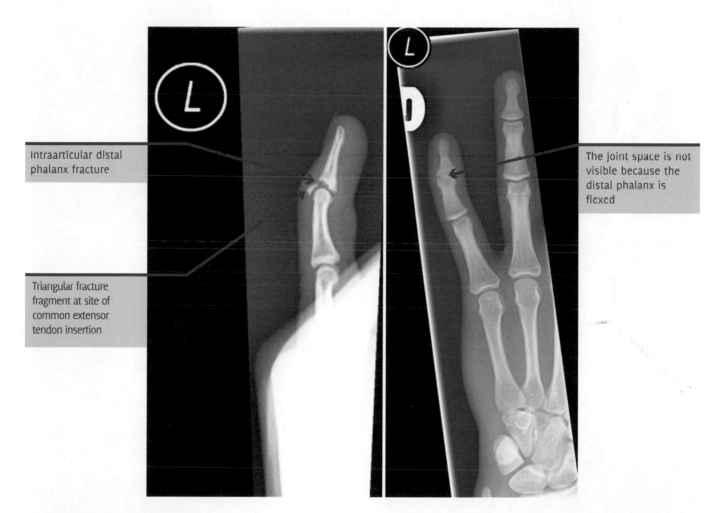

Intraarticular distal phalanx fracture

Triangular fracture fragment at site of common extensor tendon insertion

The joint space is not visible because the distal phalanx is flexed

SUMMARY AND DIFFERENTIAL

These X-rays demonstrate an avulsion fracture of the base of the distal phalanx of the 5th finger. This is consistent with a Mallet fracture. The fracture involves 50% of the articular surface.

INVESTIGATIONS AND MANAGEMENT

Appropriate analgesia should be provided.

A Mallet splint must be applied to maintain the DIPJ in fixed hyperextension. This splint should be worn at all times, 24 hours a day, and the patient should be followed up in the fracture clinic 1 week after presentation. If there is any joint subluxation on repeat X-rays, the patient may require surgery.

A 45-year-old left-hand-dominant car salesman caught his right thumb in a car door and presents to the Minor Injuries Unit. There is no significant past medical history. On examination, there is tenderness over the radial border of the thumb. Varus and valgus stress tests in full extension and 30 degrees of flexion do not reveal any laxity. Varus stress testing is painful. Distal pulses are present and sensory and motor function is preserved. The injury is closed.

AP and lateral X-rays of the right thumb are requested to assess for a fracture.

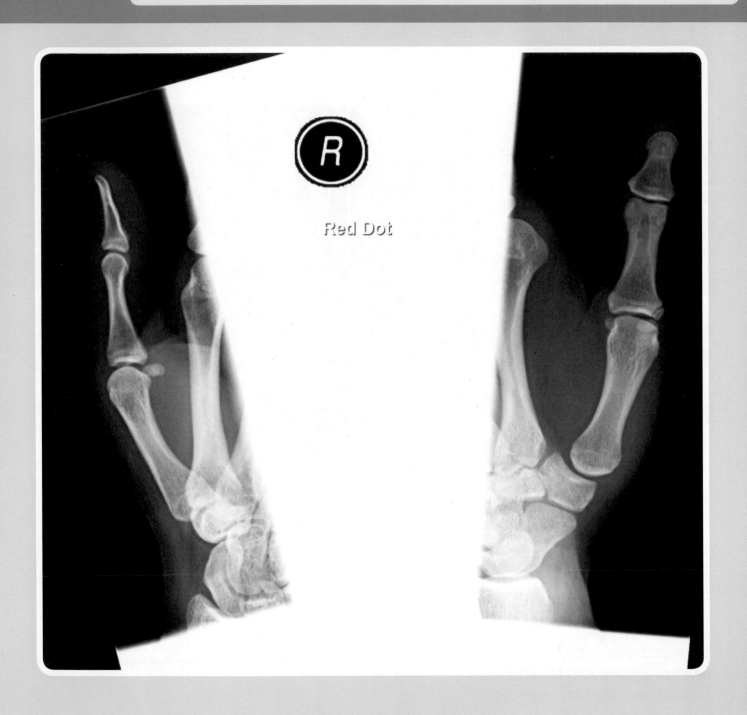

TECHNICAL INFORMATION

Patient ID: Anonymous.
Area: Right thumb.
Projection: AP and lateral.
Technical adequacy:

- Adequate coverage.
- Adequate exposure.
- The patient is not rotated.

● FRACTURE DETAILS

There is an avulsion fracture at the base of the proximal phalanx of the right thumb. The fracture involves the lateral (radial) aspect of the phalanx.

The fracture is longitudinal, simple and intraarticular.

There is ~2 mm of displacement.

There is no angulation.

There is no rotation.

There is no shortening.

● JOINTS

There is no subluxation or dislocation.

There are no loose bodies.

There is no effusion or lipohaemarthrosis.

There are no arthritic changes.

● SOFT TISSUES

There is no soft tissue swelling.

There is no surgical emphysema.

● BACKGROUND BONE

The background bone is normal.

● BONE LESIONS

There is no bone lesion present.

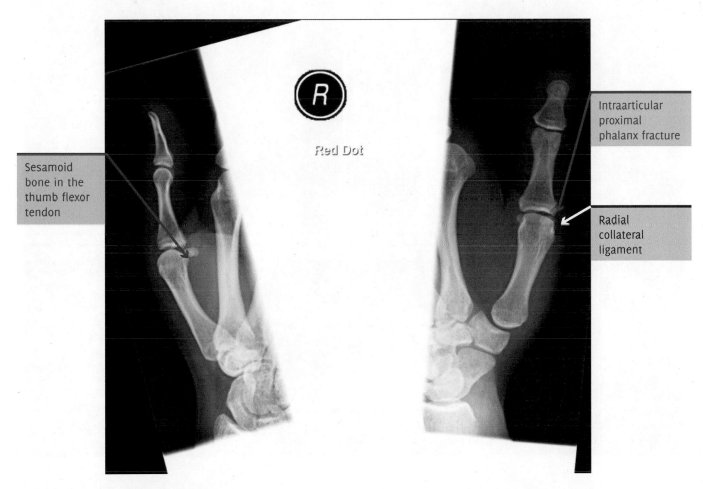

Sesamoid bone in the thumb flexor tendon

Red Dot

R

Intraarticular proximal phalanx fracture

Radial collateral ligament

SUMMARY AND DIFFERENTIAL

These X-rays demonstrate an undisplaced avulsion fracture from the radial collateral ligament, involving the base of the proximal phalanx of the thumb.

INVESTIGATIONS AND MANAGEMENT

Adequate analgesia should be provided.

A thumb spica splint should be applied and the patient referred to fracture clinic. The thumb should be splinted for 4 weeks and an early referral made to hand therapy for ongoing management.

A 21-year-old right-hand-dominant unemployed man punched someone with a partially clenched right fist. He has come to the ED the following morning. There is no significant past medical history. On examination, there is significant deformity over the knuckles of the right hand. Distal pulses are present. Sensory function is preserved but it is not possible to formally assess motor function secondary to pain. The injury is closed.

AP and oblique X-rays of the right hand are requested to assess for a fracture.

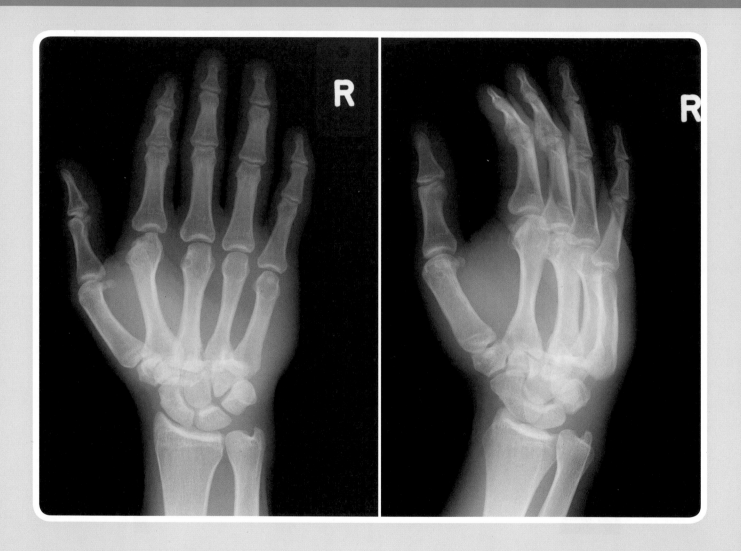

TECHNICAL INFORMATION

Patient ID: Anonymous.
Area: Right hand.
Projection: AP and oblique.
Technical adequacy:

- Adequate coverage.
- Adequate exposure.
- The patient is not rotated.

● FRACTURE DETAILS

There is no fracture.

● JOINTS

There is dislocation of the 3rd, 4th and 5th carpo-metacarpal joints with dorsal displacement of the metacarpal bases in relation to the carpal bones.

There are no loose bodies.

There is no effusion or lipohaemarthrosis.

There are no arthritic changes.

● SOFT TISSUES

There is soft tissue swelling dorsally over the hand.

There is no surgical emphysema.

● BACKGROUND BONE

The background bone is normal.

● BONE LESIONS

There is no bone lesion present.

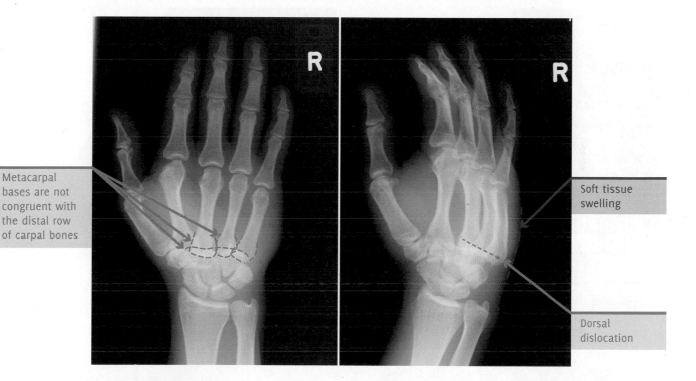

Metacarpal bases are not congruent with the distal row of carpal bones

Soft tissue swelling

Dorsal dislocation

SUMMARY AND DIFFERENTIAL

These X-rays demonstrate dorsal dislocation of the 3rd, 4th and 5th carpo-metacarpal joints.

INVESTIGATIONS AND MANAGEMENT

Appropriate analgesia should be provided.

Reduction should be attempted in the ED under sedation with orthopaedics present. A moulded back slab should be applied and repeat AP, lateral and oblique X-rays requested. A CT scan should be performed to assess for occult fracture and any residual subluxation or dislocation. Referral to orthopaedics should be made. It is likely these dislocations will be unstable and require surgical stabilization with K-wire fixation.

A 55-year-old woman developed sudden onset pain in her left little finger after only minor trauma. She has been driven to the Minor Injuries Unit by her husband. There is no significant past medical history. On examination, the patient has a painful and swollen PIPJ of her little finger. Distal pulses are present and motor and sensory function is preserved. The injury is closed.

AP and lateral X-rays of the left 5th finger are requested to assess for a fracture.

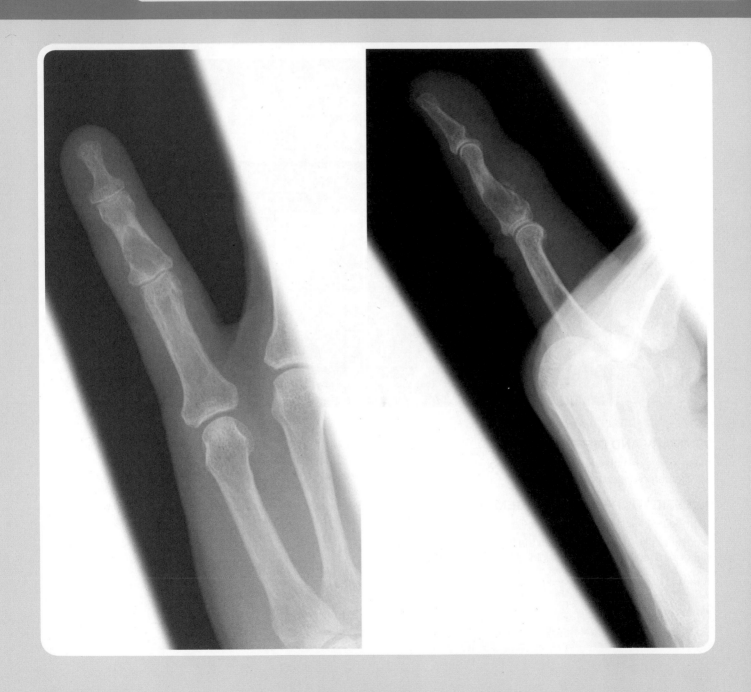

TECHNICAL INFORMATION

Patient ID: Anonymous.
Area: Left little finger.
Projection: AP and lateral.
Technical adequacy:

- Adequate coverage.
- Adequate exposure.
- The patient is not rotated.

● FRACTURE DETAILS

There is a fracture involving the middle phalanx of the little finger.

The fracture is longitudinal, simple and extraarticular.

There is no displacement.

There is no angulation.

There is no rotation.

There is no shortening.

● JOINTS

There is no subluxation or dislocation.

There are no loose bodies.

There is no effusion or lipohaemarthrosis.

There are arthritic changes with loss of joint space in the interphalangeal joints.

● SOFT TISSUES

There is no soft tissue swelling.

There is no surgical emphysema.

● BACKGROUND BONE

The background bone is normal.

● BONE LESIONS

There is a bone lesion present in the medulla of the middle phalanx.

It is lucent in appearance with some areas of calcification within the matrix.

It is not expansile.

The zone of transition is narrow with sharply defined scalloping of the adjacent cortex.

There is no bony destruction.

There is no periosteal reaction.

There is no soft tissue mass/component visible.

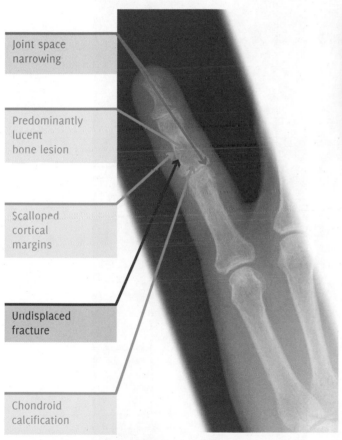

Joint space narrowing

Predominantly lucent bone lesion

Scalloped cortical margins

Undisplaced fracture

Chondroid calcification

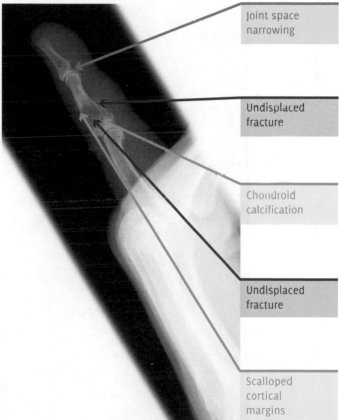

Joint space narrowing

Undisplaced fracture

Chondroid calcification

Undisplaced fracture

Scalloped cortical margins

SUMMARY AND DIFFERENTIAL

These X-rays demonstrate an undisplaced middle phalangeal fracture associated with a nonaggressive appearing bone lesion. Given the appearance of the bone lesion, the findings are consistent with a pathological fracture of an enchondroma.

INVESTIGATIONS AND MANAGEMENT

Adequate analgesia should be provided.

The finger should be splinted and a referral made to a hand surgeon. A thorough history and examination should be completed to assess for other lesions, as there are conditions of multiple enchondromas, which have a higher rate of malignant transformation. Preceding symptoms of swelling and pain before fracture would also raise the concern of transformation from enchondroma to chondrosarcoma. If there is any doubt regarding the diagnosis, consider referral to a bone tumour service.

A 12-year-old girl has fallen onto her right hand while in the playground at school. She developed immediate pain over the wrist and also sustained a laceration to the right index finger. She is brought to the ED by one of her teachers. The school nurse has applied a bandage to the wrist for comfort. There is no significant past medical history. On examination, there is full range of movement of the wrist and of all fingers. There is a graze to the index finger. On palpation, the child is tender over the distal radius, with pain on movement. Distal pulses are present and sensory and motor function is preserved.

AP and lateral X-rays of the right index finger are requested to assess for a foreign body.

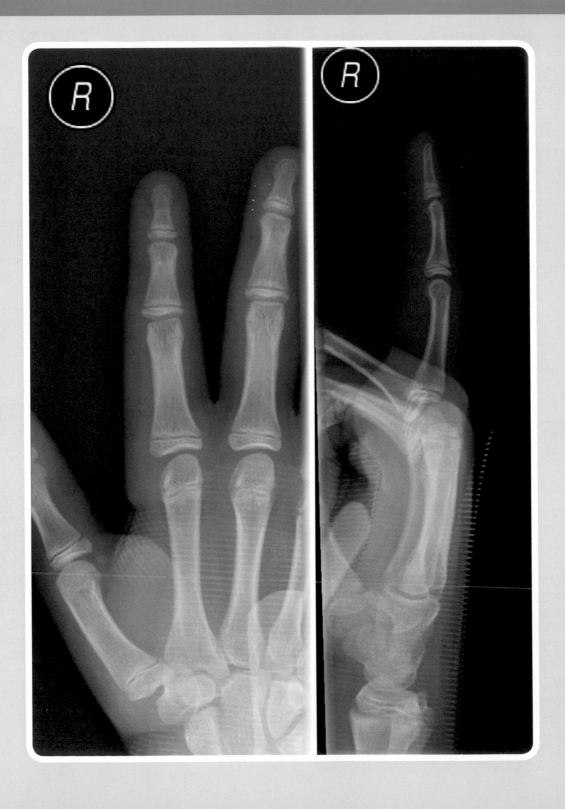

TECHNICAL INFORMATION

Patient ID: Anonymous.
Area: Right index finger.
Projection: AP and lateral.
Technical adequacy:

- Adequate coverage.
- Adequate exposure.
- The patient is not rotated.

● FRACTURE DETAILS

There is a possible subtle fracture involving the right distal radius. It is visible only on the lateral X-ray.

The fracture is buckle-type, simple and extraarticular.

There is no displacement.

There is no angulation.

There is no rotation.

There is no shortening.

● JOINTS

There is no subluxation or dislocation.

There are no loose bodies.

There is no effusion or lipohaemarthrosis.

There are no arthritic changes.

● SOFT TISSUES

There is no radio-opaque foreign body.

There is no soft tissue swelling.

There is no surgical emphysema.

● BACKGROUND BONE

The background bone is normal.

● BONE LESIONS

There is no bone lesion present.

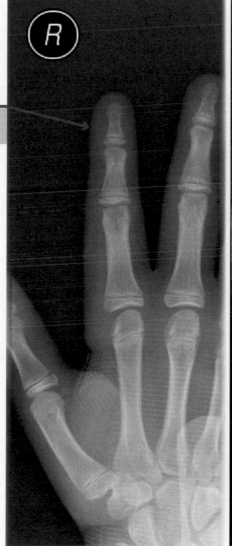

No radio-opaque foreign body

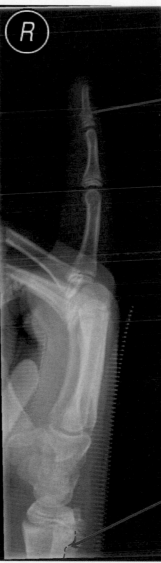

No radio-opaque foreign body

Subtle distal radial buckle fracture

SUMMARY AND DIFFERENTIAL

These X-rays suggest a buckle fracture of the right distal radius although these are not wrist X-rays. No radio-opaque foreign body is visible.

INVESTIGATIONS AND MANAGEMENT

Appropriate analgesia should be provided.

The wrist should be imaged with complete views to assess the fracture and identify any other associated injuries.

Depending on the wrist imaging, management may be with a moulded back slab or splint and the patient should be referred to fracture clinic.

An 8-year-old boy fell off the monkey bars in the park. He landed on an outstretched right hand and is brought to the ED by his parents. There is no significant past medical history. On examination, there is swelling around the right wrist and all movements of the wrist are painful. There is no gross deformity, distal pulses are present and sensory and motor function is preserved.

AP and lateral X-rays of the right wrist are requested to assess for fracture.

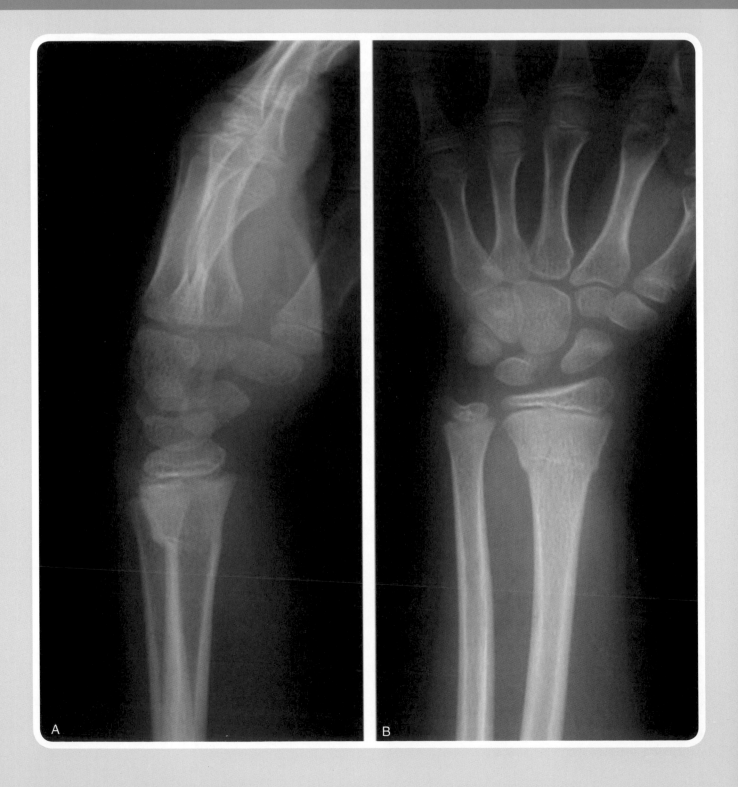

A   B

TECHNICAL INFORMATION

Patient ID: Anonymous.
Area: Right wrist.
Projection: AP and lateral.
Technical adequacy:

- Adequate coverage.
- Adequate exposure.
- The patient is not rotated.

● FRACTURE DETAILS

There is a fracture involving the distal radius.

It is transverse, simple and extraarticular.

There is no displacement.

Minimal dorsal angulation is present.

There is no rotation.

There is no shortening.

● JOINTS

There is no subluxation or dislocation.

There are no loose bodies.

There is no effusion or lipohaemarthrosis.

There are no arthritic changes.

● SOFT TISSUES

There is no soft tissue swelling.

There is no surgical emphysema.

● BACKGROUND BONE

The background bone is normal.

● BONE LESIONS

There is no bone lesion present.

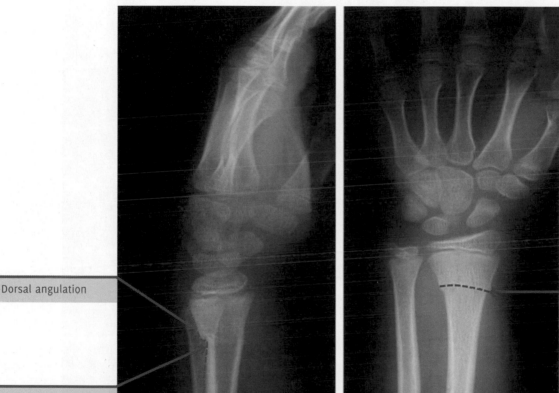

Dorsal angulation

Distal radial buckle fracture

Distal radial buckle fracture

A

B

SUMMARY AND DIFFERENTIAL

These X-rays demonstrate a paediatric distal radius fracture with minimal dorsal angulation. This pattern of fracture is called a *buckle fracture*. The periosteum lining the bones is intact and so the fracture will heal well without surgical intervention.

INVESTIGATIONS AND MANAGEMENT

Appropriate analgesia should be provided.

An elasticated wrist splint should be provided with advice to initially elevate the limb and keep fingers moving to reduce the swelling. A buckle fracture leaflet should be provided. The patient should be advised to wear the splint the majority of the time, except for washing. The patient can remove the splint after 3 weeks and begin gentle range of movement exercises. Return to sport usually takes a further 3 weeks.

A 6-year-old girl fell from a trampoline onto her outstretched left hand. She is brought to the ED by her parents as she is in significant pain, and they think the wrist looks swollen. There is no significant past medical history. On examination, there is a visible deformity of the left wrist. There is marked swelling and bruising around the wrist. All movements are painful. Distal pulses are present and sensory and motor function is preserved. The injury is closed.

AP and lateral X-rays of the left wrist are requested to assess for a fracture.

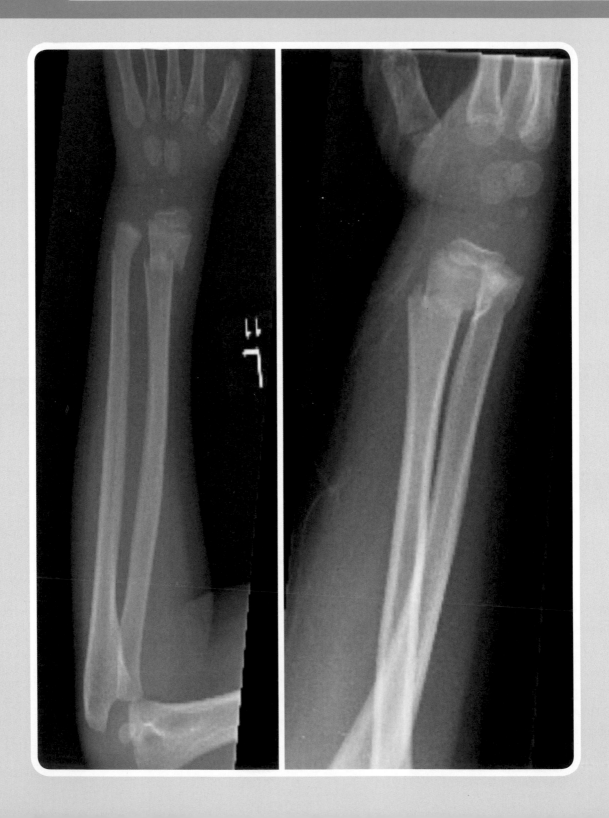

TECHNICAL INFORMATION

Patient ID: Anonymous.
Area: Left wrist.
Projection: AP and lateral.
Technical adequacy:

- Adequate coverage.
- Adequate exposure.
- The lateral X-ray is not a true lateral.

● FRACTURE DETAILS

There is a fracture involving the metaphysis of the distal radius.

It is transverse, simple and extraarticular.

There is dorsal and lateral (radial direction) displacement of approximately 5 mm.

There is also dorsal angulation of approximately 20 degrees.

There is no rotation.

There is minimal shortening of the radius.

There is a fracture involving the metaphysis of the distal ulna.

The fracture is transverse, simple and extraarticular.

There is no translational displacement.

Minor lateral (radial direction) angulation is present.

There is no rotation.

There is no shortening.

● JOINTS

There is no subluxation or dislocation of the distal radioulnar joint or elbow joint, although the latter has not been adequately assessed.

There are no loose bodies.

There is no effusion or lipohaemarthrosis.

There are no arthritic changes.

● SOFT TISSUES

Minor soft tissue swelling is present.

There is no surgical emphysema.

● BACKGROUND BONE

The background bone is normal.

● BONE LESIONS

There is no bone lesion present.

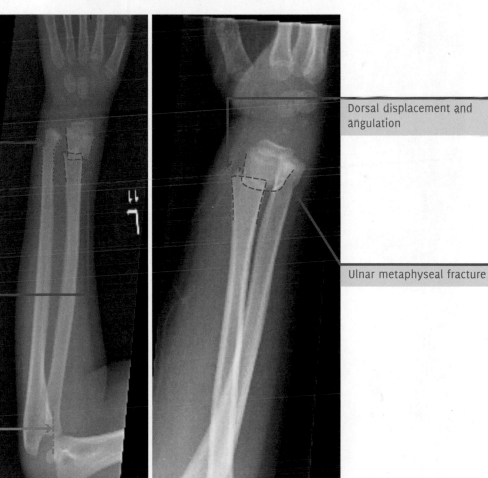

Ulnar metaphyseal fracture with minor lateral (radial) angulation

Lateral (radial) displacement

Normal radiocapitellar alignment

Dorsal displacement and angulation

Ulnar metaphyseal fracture

SUMMARY AND DIFFERENTIAL

The X-rays demonstrate fractures of the distal radius and ulna. There is displacement, which is likely underestimated on the oblique lateral X-ray.

INVESTIGATIONS AND MANAGEMENT

Advice regarding analgesia should be provided. A below-elbow back slab should be applied with repeat X-rays in back slab. These will likely demonstrate that there is significant dorsal displacement. The patient requires referral to orthopaedics, who will consider a manipulation under anaesthetic in theatre with or without the use of K wires.

A 9-year-old girl has fallen onto her outstretched left hand. She tripped on the pavement on the way to school. She is now complaining of pain in her wrist and has been brought to the Minor Injuries Unit by her parents. There is no significant past medical history. On examination, there is pain around the wrist. Movement is present but painful. Distal pulses are present and sensory and motor function is preserved. The injury is closed.

AP and lateral X-rays of the left wrist are requested to assess for fracture.

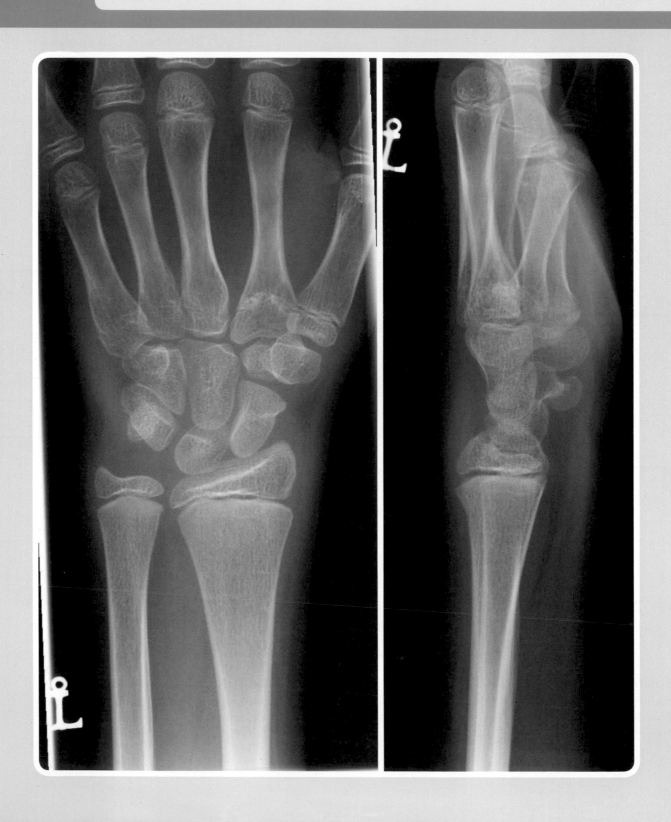

TECHNICAL INFORMATION

Patient ID: Anonymous.
Area: Left wrist.
Projection: AP and lateral.
Technical adequacy:

- Adequate coverage.
- Adequate exposure.
- The patient is not rotated.

● FRACTURE DETAILS

There is a fracture involving the distal radial metaphysis.

The fracture is transverse, simple and extraarticular.

There is no displacement.

There is no angulation.

There is no rotation.

There is no shortening.

● JOINTS

There is no subluxation or dislocation.

There are no loose bodies.

There is no effusion or lipohaemarthrosis.

There are no arthritic changes.

● SOFT TISSUES

There is no soft tissue swelling.

There is no surgical emphysema.

● BACKGROUND BONE

The background bone is normal.

● BONE LESIONS

There is no bone lesion present.

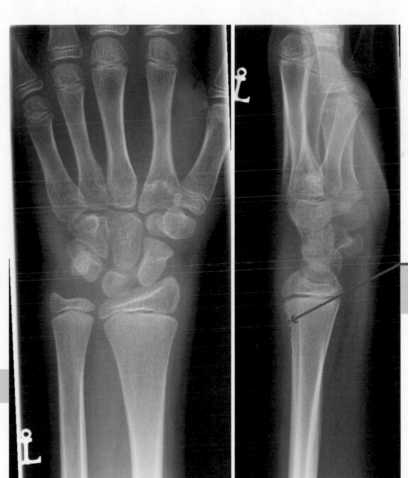

Normal appearances on the AP view

Subtle radial metaphyseal buckle fracture on visible on the lateral radiograph

SUMMARY AND DIFFERENTIAL

The lateral X-ray demonstrates a minimally displaced distal radius buckle fracture.

INVESTIGATIONS AND MANAGEMENT

Adequate analgesia should be provided.

An elasticated wrist splint should be provided with advice to initially elevate the limb and keep fingers moving to reduce the swelling. A buckle fracture leaflet should be provided.

The patient should be advised to wear the splint the majority of the time, except for washing. The patient can remove the splint after 3 weeks and begin gentle range of movement exercises. Return to sport usually takes a further 3 weeks.

A nonbinary 55-year-old presents to the ED. They suffered a fall whilst ice skating with their spouse. They describe landing on their outstretched right hand. They have severe pain in their right wrist, which they are unable to move. There is no significant past medical history. On examination, there is swelling over the wrist, with tenderness on palpation. Distal pulses are present and sensory and motor function is preserved. The injury is closed.

AP and lateral X-rays of the right wrist are requested to assess for a fracture.

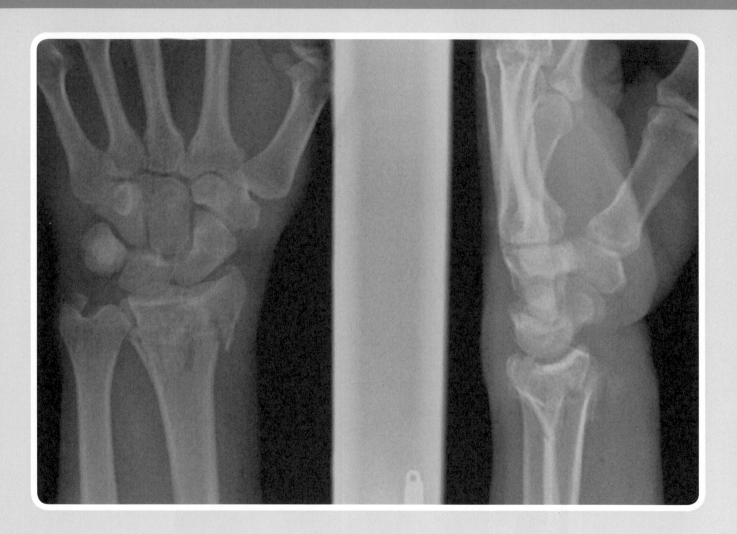

TECHNICAL INFORMATION

Patient ID: Anonymous.
Area: Right wrist.
Projection: AP and lateral.
Technical adequacy:

- Adequate coverage.
- Adequate exposure.
- The patient is not rotated.

● FRACTURE DETAILS

There is a fracture involving the distal radius.

The fracture is transverse, comminuted and intraarticular.

Radial (lateral) displacement, posterior displacement and dorsal (posterior) angulation is present.

There is no rotation.

There is shortening present.

There is a fracture involving the ulna styloid.

The fracture is transverse, simple and intraarticular.

There is radial (lateral) displacement present.

There is no angulation.

There is no rotation.

● JOINTS

There is subluxation and dislocation.

There are no loose bodies.

There is no effusion or lipohaemarthrosis.

There are no arthritic changes.

● SOFT TISSUES

There is soft tissue swelling dorsally.

There is no surgical emphysema.

● BACKGROUND BONE

The background bone is normal.

● BONE LESIONS

There is no bone lesion present.

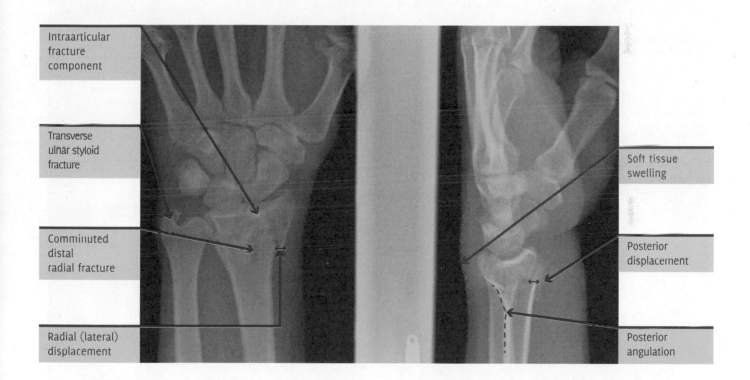

Intraarticular fracture component

Transverse ulnar styloid fracture

Comminuted distal radial fracture

Radial (lateral) displacement

Soft tissue swelling

Posterior displacement

Posterior angulation

SUMMARY AND DIFFERENTIAL

These X-rays demonstrate a right distal radial intraarticular fracture with dorsal angulation. There is an associated ulnar styloid fracture.

INVESTIGATIONS AND MANAGEMENT

Analgesia should be provided.

The fracture should undergo closed reduction in the ED under one of many suitable techniques including sedation, haematoma block or Biers block. A moulded back slab should be applied. Postreduction X-rays should be taken.

A referral should be made to orthopaedics who may consider surgical fixation depending on the patient and the postreduction X-rays.

A 71-year-old woman has come in to the ED. She tripped over the curb and describes landing on her outstretched left hand. Her left wrist is now very painful. She has a past medical history of osteoporosis. On examination, the wrist is visibly deformed, with associated tenderness and swelling. Distal pulses are present and sensory and motor function is preserved. The injury is closed.

AP and lateral X-rays of the left wrist are requested to assess for a fracture.

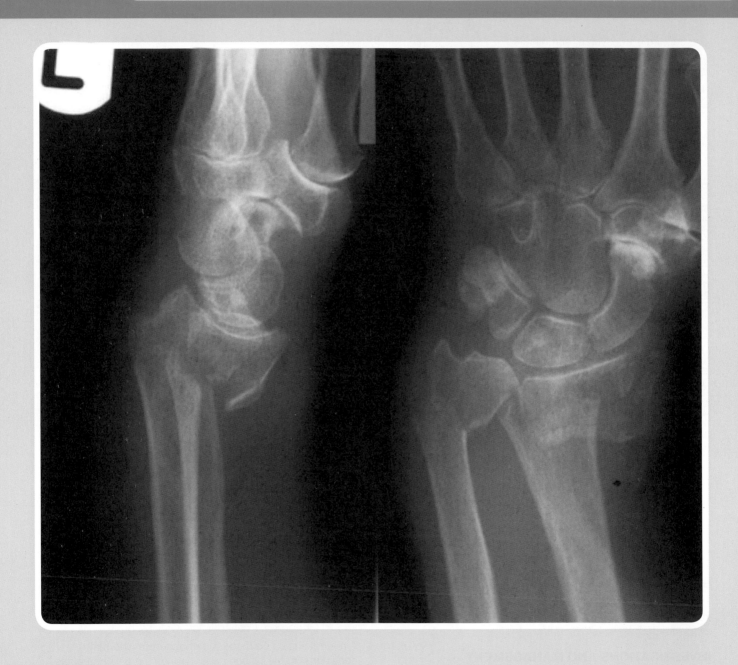

TECHNICAL INFORMATION

Patient ID: Anonymous.
Area: Left wrist.
Projection: AP and lateral.
Technical adequacy:

- Adequate coverage.
- Adequate exposure.
- The patient is not rotated.

● FRACTURE DETAILS

There is a fracture involving the distal radius.

The fracture is transverse, simple and intraarticular.

There is radial (lateral) displacement, volar (anterior) angulation and shortening present.

There is no rotation.

There is a fracture involving the distal ulna.

The fracture is transverse, simple and extraarticular.

There is radial (lateral) displacement along with volar (anterior) and radial (lateral) angulation.

There is no rotation.

There is no shortening.

● JOINTS

There is no subluxation or dislocation.

There are no loose bodies.

There is no effusion or lipohaemarthrosis.

There are arthritic changes at the scaphotrapezium-trapezoid joints, with loss of joint space and subchondral sclerosis.

● SOFT TISSUES

There is soft tissue swelling on the distal ulnar side of the wrist.

There is no surgical emphysema.

● BACKGROUND BONE

The background bone is osteopenic.

● BONE LESIONS

There is no bone lesion present.

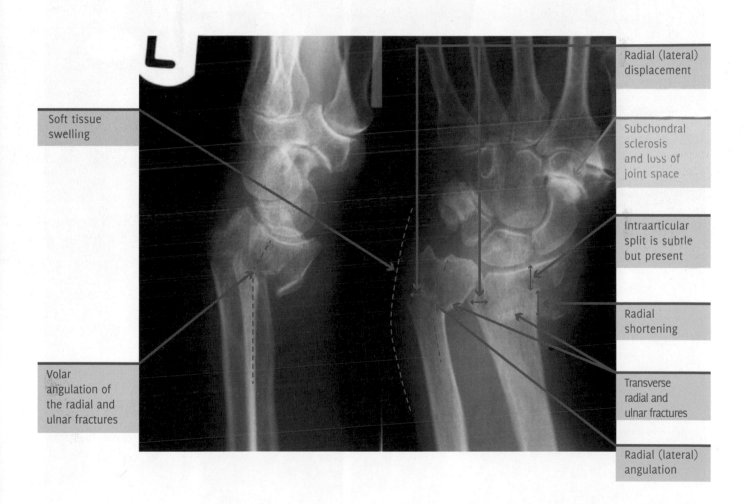

Soft tissue swelling

Volar angulation of the radial and ulnar fractures

Radial (lateral) displacement

Subchondral sclerosis and loss of joint space

Intraarticular split is subtle but present

Radial shortening

Transverse radial and ulnar fractures

Radial (lateral) angulation

SUMMARY AND DIFFERENTIAL

Both X-rays demonstrate an intraarticular distal radius fracture with volar angulation and an associated ulnar fracture.

INVESTIGATIONS AND MANAGEMENT

Analgesia should be provided.

The fracture should undergo closed reduction in the ED under one of many suitable techniques including sedation, haematoma block or Biers block. A moulded back slab should be applied. Postreduction X-rays should be taken.

A referral should be made to orthopaedics who will consider surgical fixation.

A 76-year-old woman has been brought to hospital by her husband after she tripped down the stairs at home. She describes landing on her outstretched right hand. She is complaining of pain in the wrist and states that it looks abnormal. There is no significant past medical history. On examination, there is an obviously deformed forearm, with tenderness over the wrist. Distal pulses are present and motor and sensory function is preserved. The injury is closed.

AP and lateral X-rays of the right wrist are requested to assess for a fracture.

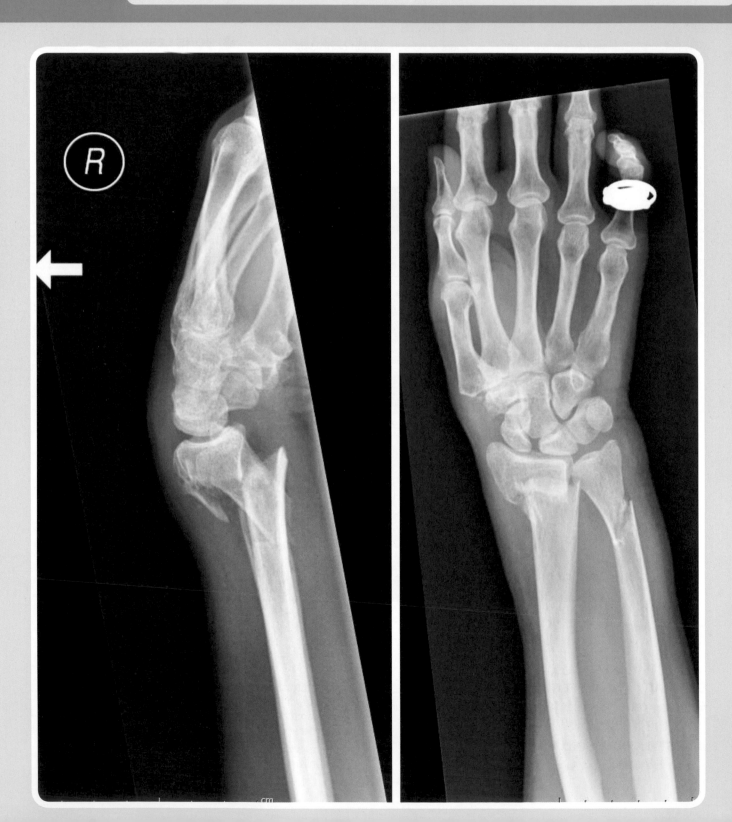

TECHNICAL INFORMATION

Patient ID: Anonymous.
Area: Right wrist.
Projection: AP and lateral.
Technical adequacy:

- Adequate coverage.
- Adequate exposure.
- The patient is not rotated.

● FRACTURE DETAILS

There is a fracture involving the distal radius.

The fracture is transverse, comminuted and extraarticular.

There is marked dorsal (posterior) and mild radial (lateral) displacement along with dorsal (posterior) angulation.

There is shortening.

There is no rotation.

There is a fracture involving the distal ulna.

The fracture is oblique, simple and extraarticular with marked dorsal (posterior) angulation.

There is no translational displacement.

There is no rotation.

There is no shortening.

● JOINTS

There is no subluxation or dislocation.

There are no loose bodies.

There is no effusion or lipohaemarthrosis.

There are no arthritic changes.

● SOFT TISSUES

There is soft tissue swelling.

There is no surgical emphysema.

● BACKGROUND BONE

The background bone is normal.

● BONE LESIONS

There is no bone lesion present.

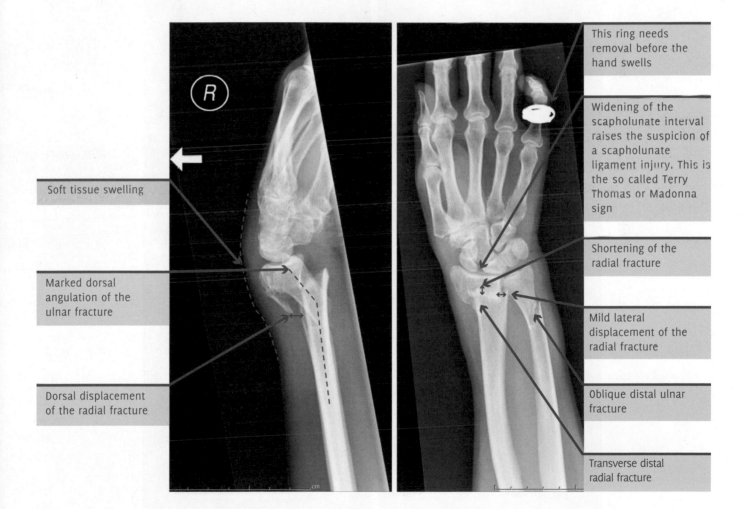

Soft tissue swelling

Marked dorsal angulation of the ulnar fracture

Dorsal displacement of the radial fracture

This ring needs removal before the hand swells

Widening of the scapholunate interval raises the suspicion of a scapholunate ligament injury. This is the so called Terry Thomas or Madonna sign

Shortening of the radial fracture

Mild lateral displacement of the radial fracture

Oblique distal ulnar fracture

Transverse distal radial fracture

SUMMARY AND DIFFERENTIAL

Both X-rays demonstrate a dorsally angulated and displaced distal radial fracture with an associated distal ulna shaft fracture.

INVESTIGATIONS AND MANAGEMENT

Analgesia should be provided.

The fracture should undergo closed reduction in the ED under one of many suitable techniques including sedation, haematoma block or Biers block. A moulded back slab should be applied. Postreduction X-rays should be taken. A referral should be made to orthopaedics who may consider surgical fixation.

A 9-year-old boy has been brought to the ED by his mother. He was playing football in the playground at school when he tripped. He describes landing on his outstretched right hand. His hand is very painful and visibly deformed. There is no significant past medical history. On examination, there is a clear deformity of the right wrist, which is painful. The radial pulse is not palpable, although the hand is pink and perfused. Sensory and motor function is initially felt to be preserved but after closer examination, the child states the fingers feel sparkly. The injury is closed.

AP and lateral X-rays of the right wrist are requested to assess for a fracture.

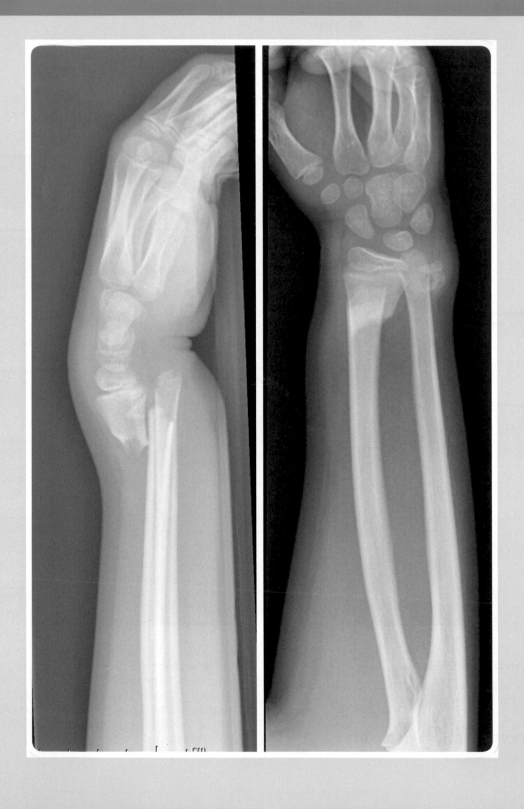

TECHNICAL INFORMATION

Patient ID: Anonymous.
Area: Right wrist.
Projection: AP and lateral.
Technical adequacy:

- Adequate coverage.
- Adequate exposure.
- The patient is not rotated.

● FRACTURE DETAILS

There is a fracture involving the distal radial metaphysis.

The fracture is transverse, simple and extraarticular.

There is complete dorsal (posterior) displacement and dorsal (posterior) angulation.

There is marked shortening.

There is no rotation.

There is a fracture involving the distal ulnar metaphysis.

The fracture is transverse, simple and extraarticular.

There is complete dorsal (posterior) displacement and dorsal (posterior) angulation.

There is marked shortening.

There is no rotation.

● JOINTS

There is no subluxation or dislocation.

There are no loose bodies.

There is no effusion or lipohaemarthrosis.

There are no arthritic changes.

● SOFT TISSUES

There is soft tissue swelling.

There is no surgical emphysema.

● BACKGROUND BONE

The background bone is normal.

● BONE LESIONS

There is no bone lesion present.

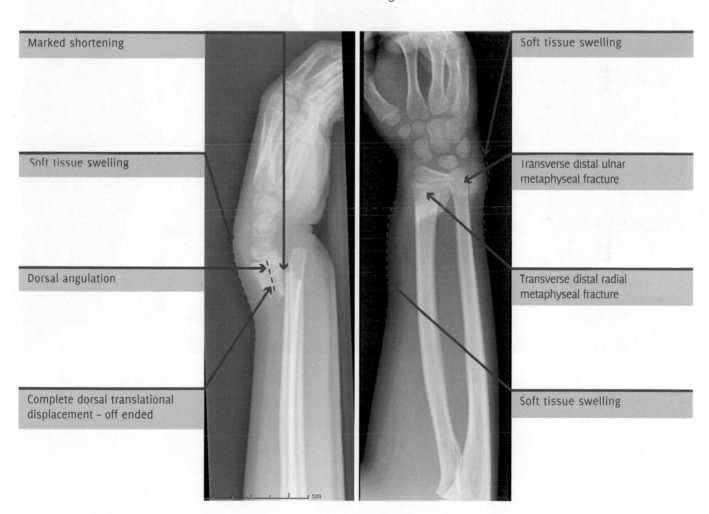

Marked shortening

Soft tissue swelling

Dorsal angulation

Complete dorsal translational displacement – off ended

Soft tissue swelling

Transverse distal ulnar metaphyseal fracture

Transverse distal radial metaphyseal fracture

Soft tissue swelling

SUMMARY AND DIFFERENTIAL

Both X-rays demonstrate right distal radial and ulnar metaphyseal fractures with complete dorsal displacement and marked shortening. There is vascular and sensory compromise.

INVESTIGATIONS AND MANAGEMENT

Analgesia should be provided.

Because of the lack of a pulse, the patient will need to be urgently referred to orthopaedics. Further intervention will include closed reduction in theatre under X-ray with the likely use of supplementary fixation using K wires. Following reduction, serial examinations of pulses and sensory and motor function are required. As the hand was pink before reduction, it is most likely that pulses and sensory function will return, but if there is any concern then an early vascular opinion should be sought.

An 88-year-old woman with dementia is brought to the ED from her nursing home. She had an unwitnessed fall in the home. Staff noticed a deformity of the left wrist and called an ambulance. The only significant medical history is Alzheimer disease. On examination, there is a visibly deformed left wrist that is tender on palpation, but distal pulses and motor and sensory function are preserved. The injury is closed.

AP and lateral X-rays of the left wrist are requested to assess for a fracture.

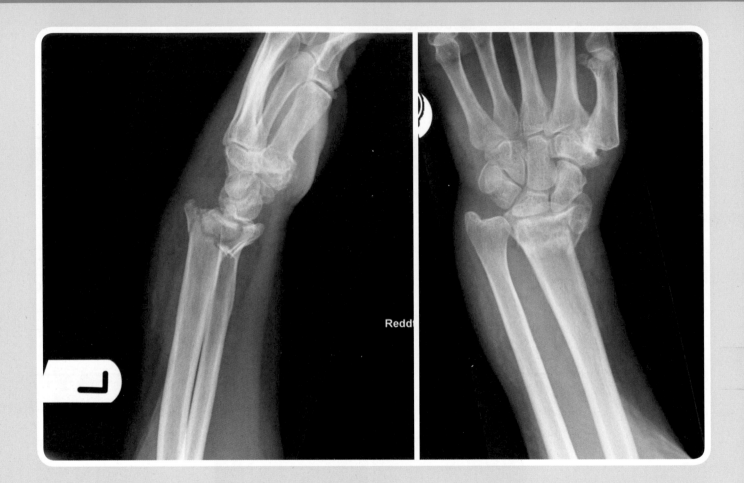

TECHNICAL INFORMATION

Patient ID: Anonymous.
Area: Left wrist.
Projection: AP and lateral.
Technical adequacy:

- Adequate coverage.
- Adequate exposure.
- The patient is slightly rotated on the lateral view.

● FRACTURE DETAILS

There is a fracture involving the distal radius.

The fracture is transverse, comminuted and intraarticular.

Volar (anterior) angulation and shortening are observed.

There is no displacement.

There is no rotation.

● JOINTS

There is no subluxation or dislocation.

There are no loose bodies.

There is no effusion or lipohaemarthrosis.

There are arthritic changes affecting the 1st carpo-metacarpal joint, with loss of joint space and subchondral sclerosis.

● SOFT TISSUES

There is soft tissue swelling present.

There is no surgical emphysema.

● BACKGROUND BONE

The background bone is normal.

● BONE LESIONS

There is no bone lesion present.

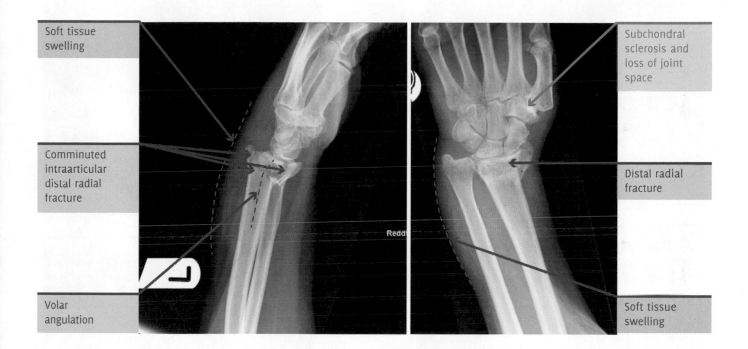

Soft tissue swelling

Comminuted intraarticular distal radial fracture

Volar angulation

Subchondral sclerosis and loss of joint space

Distal radial fracture

Soft tissue swelling

SUMMARY AND DIFFERENTIAL

Both X-rays demonstrate an intraarticular distal radial fracture with volar angulation.

INVESTIGATIONS AND MANAGEMENT

Analgesia should be provided.

Because of the patient's functional status (dementia, nursing home resident), she would most likely be managed nonoperatively with reduction in the ED and a moulded cast for 6 weeks. In a fitter, more high-demand patient, a referral would be made to orthopaedics to consider surgical fixation.

A 27-year-old woman presents to the ED. She slipped on the wet floor when getting out of the bath and landed on her outstretched right hand. She now complains of a very painful and bruised hand. There is no significant past medical history. On examination, the wrist is tender, and all movements are very painful. Distal pulses are present and sensory and motor function are preserved. The injury is closed.

AP and lateral X-rays of the right wrist are requested to assess for a fracture.

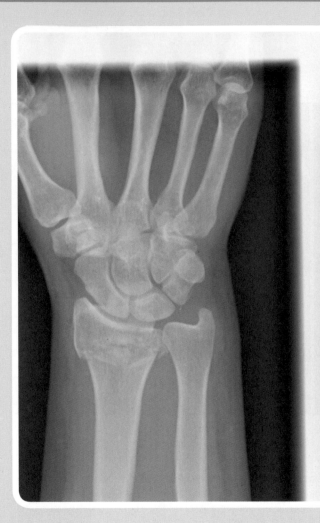
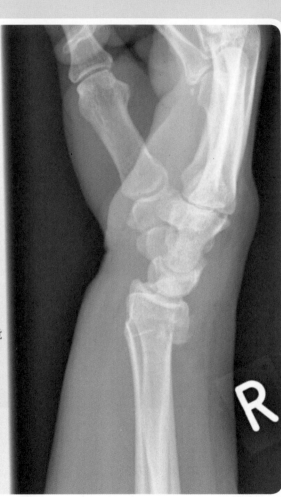

TECHNICAL INFORMATION

Patient ID: Anonymous.
Area: Right wrist.
Projection: AP and lateral.
Technical adequacy:

- Adequate coverage.
- Adequate exposure.
- The patient is not rotated.

● FRACTURE DETAILS

There is a fracture involving the distal radius.

The fracture is transverse, simple and extraarticular.

Dorsal angulation and shortening are present.

There is no displacement.

There is no rotation.

● JOINTS

There is no subluxation or dislocation.

There are no loose bodies.

There is no effusion or lipohaemarthrosis.

There are no arthritic changes.

● SOFT TISSUES

There is no soft tissue swelling.

There is no surgical emphysema.

● BACKGROUND BONE

The background bone is normal.

● BONE LESIONS

There is no bone lesion present.

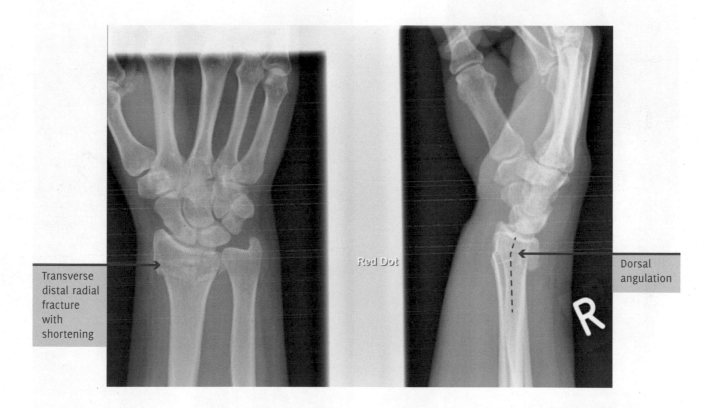

Transverse distal radial fracture with shortening

Red Dot

Dorsal angulation

R

SUMMARY AND DIFFERENTIAL

Both X-rays demonstrate a dorsally angulated distal radius fracture. This would be classified as a Colles fracture.

INVESTIGATIONS AND MANAGEMENT

Analgesia should be provided.

The fracture should undergo closed reduction in the ED under one of many suitable techniques including sedation, haematoma block or Biers block. A moulded back slab should be applied. Postreduction X-rays should be taken. If displacement remains after reduction, a referral should be made to orthopaedics who may consider reduction under general anaesthetic and K-wire fixation. If the reduction is adequate, then serial X-rays are required to ensure that there is no redisplacement.

A 53-year-old man attends the ED complaining of pain in his right hand. He slipped earlier in the day in a muddy field, landing on his outstretched right hand. There is no significant past medical history. On examination, there is tenderness over the wrist and in the anatomical snuffbox. All movements of the wrist are painful. Distal pulses are present and motor and sensory function are preserved. The injury is closed.

AP and lateral X-rays of the right wrist are requested to assess for a fracture.

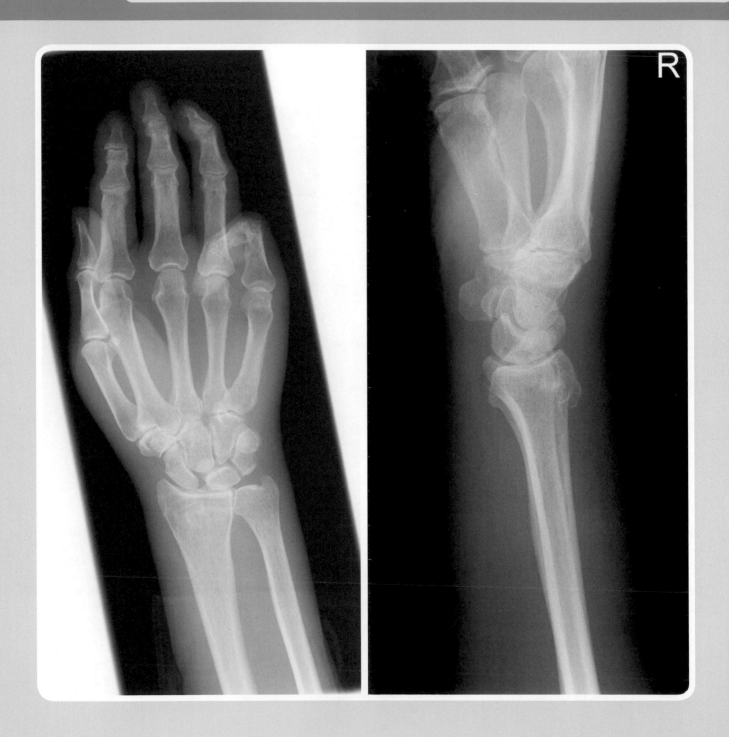

TECHNICAL INFORMATION

Patient ID: Anonymous.
Area: Right wrist.
Projection: AP and lateral.
Technical adequacy:

- Adequate coverage.
- Adequate exposure.
- The patient is not rotated.

● FRACTURE DETAILS

There is an irregularity of the distal dorsal radial cortex, consistent with a fracture.

The fracture is transverse, simple and extraarticular.

There is no displacement.

There is no angulation.

There is no rotation.

There is no shortening.

● JOINTS

There is widening of the scapholunate gap, which is consistent with scapholunate dissociation.

There are no loose bodies.

There is no effusion or lipohaemarthrosis.

There are no arthritic changes.

● SOFT TISSUES

There is no soft tissue swelling.

There is no surgical emphysema.

● BACKGROUND BONE

The background bone is normal.

● BONE LESIONS

There is no bone lesion present.

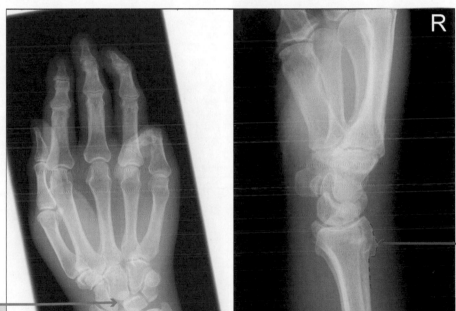

Widened scapholunate space. This is known as the Terry Thomas or Madonna sign.

Irregular dorsal distal radial cortex

SUMMARY AND DIFFERENTIAL

Both X-rays demonstrate a right undisplaced distal radius fracture. There is also dissociation of the scaphoid and lunate.

INVESTIGATIONS AND MANAGEMENT

Advice regarding analgesia should be provided.

The scapholunate dissociation requires referral to a plastic or hand surgeon for an opinion. Treatment may include acute scapholunate ligament repair. The fracture will require a below-elbow cast for 4 weeks.

A 37-year-old male presents to the ED. He was cycling downhill at approximately 30 mph when he lost control of his bike. He landed on an outstretched left hand. He is complaining of pain in his hand and has tingling in the middle and ring fingers. There is no significant past medical history. On examination, there is tenderness over the carpus, with swelling over the wrist. There is altered sensation in the distribution of the median nerve. Distal pulses are present and sensory and motor function is otherwise preserved. The injury is closed.

AP and lateral X-rays of the left wrist are requested to assess for a fracture.

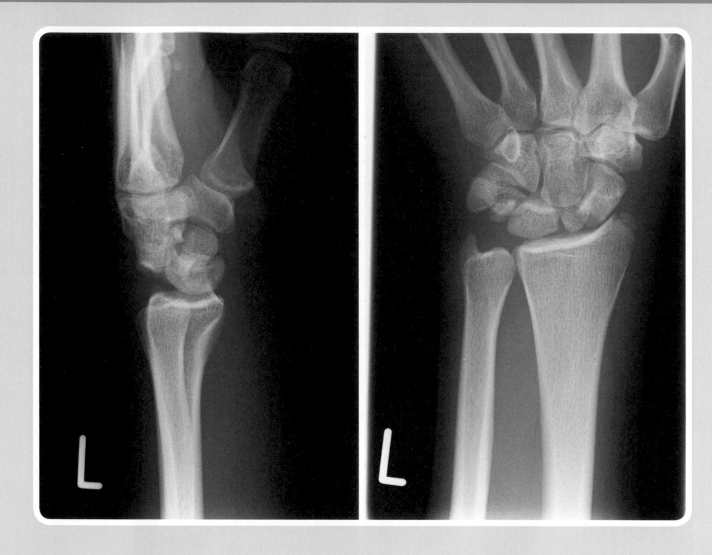

TECHNICAL INFORMATION

Patient ID: Anonymous.
Area: Left wrist.
Projection: AP/lateral.
Technical adequacy:

- Adequate coverage.
- Adequate exposure.
- The patient is not rotated.

● FRACTURE DETAILS

There is a fracture involving the radial styloid.

The fracture is oblique, simple and intraarticular.

There is minimal displacement.

There is no angulation.

There is no rotation.

There is no shortening.

There is a fracture of the proximal pole of the scaphoid.

The fracture is oblique, simple and intraarticular.

There is minimal displacement.

There is angulation.

There is rotation.

There is no shortening.

● JOINTS

The lunate is normally aligned with the distal radius, while the capitate and other carpal bones are dislocated dorsally (posteriorly).

There are no loose bodies.

There is no effusion or lipohaemarthrosis.

There are no arthritic changes.

● SOFT TISSUES

There is no soft tissue swelling.

There is no surgical emphysema.

● BACKGROUND BONE

The background bone is normal.

● BONE LESIONS

There is no bone lesion present.

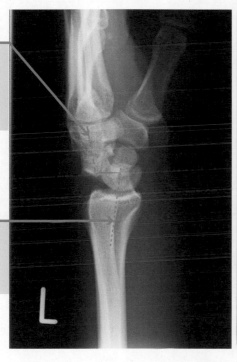

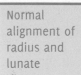

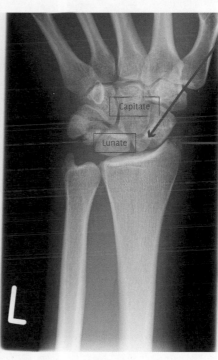

Dorsal dislocation of the capitate and other carpal bones

Normal alignment of radius and lunate

Proximal pole fracture of the scaphoid

Capitate

Lunate

Undisplaced radial styloid fracture

SUMMARY AND DIFFERENTIAL

Both X-rays demonstrate a left trans-scaphoid perilunate dislocation. There is also an associated radial styloid fracture. The clinical features suggest compromise of the median nerve.

INVESTIGATIONS AND MANAGEMENT

Analgesia should be provided.

An emergency referral should be made to an orthopaedic surgeon who may consider closed reduction, application of a moulded back slab and acute carpal tunnel decompression.

For definitive treatment, the patient will need referral to a hand or plastic surgeon for open reduction, ligament repair and scaphoid fracture fixation.

A 34-year-old woman attends the ED. She fell whilst walking upstairs and landed on her left outstretched arm. She has pain in her wrist and her partner is worried that she may have broken it. There is no significant past medical history. On examination, there is tenderness over the left wrist with movements possible but painful. Distal pulses are present and sensory and motor function are preserved. The injury is closed.

AP and lateral X-rays of the left wrist are requested to assess for a fracture.

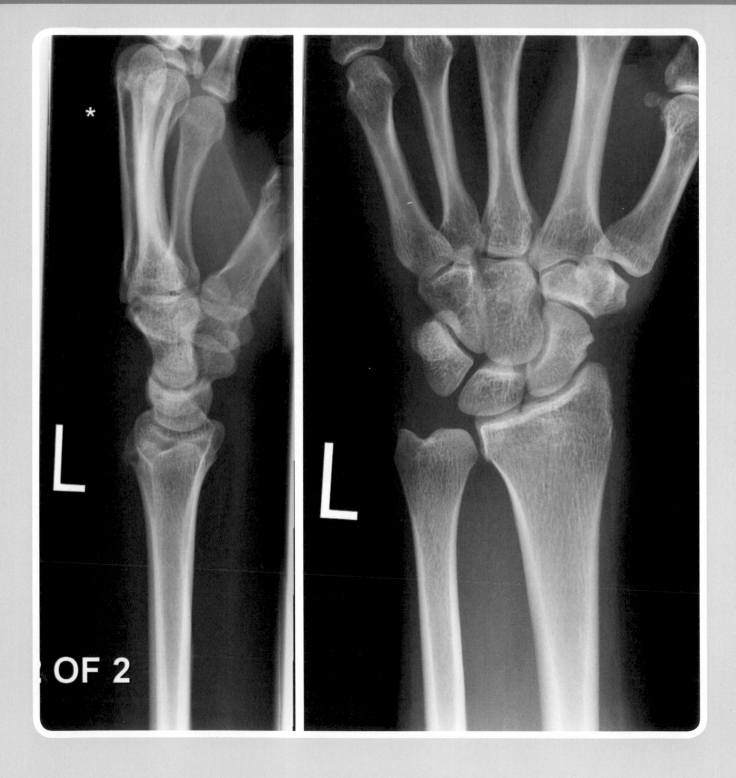

TECHNICAL INFORMATION

Patient ID: Anonymous.
Area: Left wrist.
Projection: AP and lateral.
Technical adequacy:

- Adequate coverage.
- Adequate exposure.
- The patient is not rotated.

● FRACTURE DETAILS

There is an irregularity of the distal dorsal radial cortex, which is consistent with a fracture. On the AP X-ray, there is a line extending into the articular surface.

The fracture is simple and intraarticular.

There is no displacement.

There is no angulation.

There is no rotation.

There is no shortening.

● JOINTS

There is no subluxation or dislocation.

There are no loose bodies.

There is no effusion or lipohaemarthrosis.

There are no arthritic changes.

● SOFT TISSUES

There is no soft tissue swelling.

There is no surgical emphysema.

● BACKGROUND BONE

The background bone is normal.

● BONE LESIONS

There is no bone lesion present.

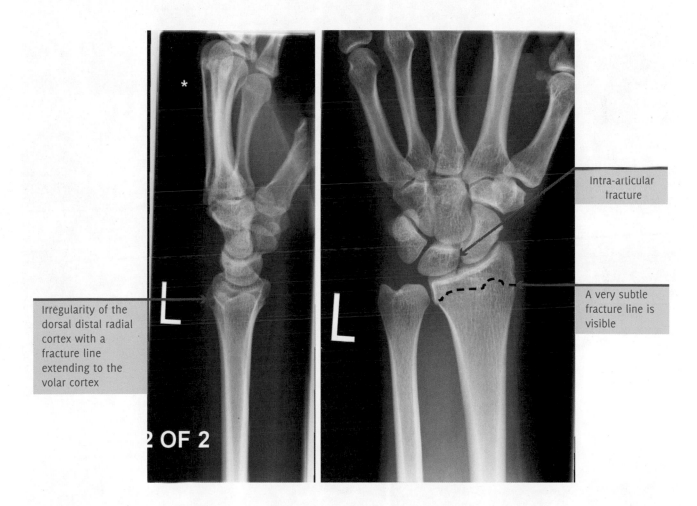

Irregularity of the dorsal distal radial cortex with a fracture line extending to the volar cortex

Intra-articular fracture

A very subtle fracture line is visible

SUMMARY AND DIFFERENTIAL

The lateral X-ray demonstrates an undisplaced intraarticular left distal radius fracture.

INVESTIGATIONS AND MANAGEMENT

Analgesia should be provided.

A CT scan should be performed to assess for the degree of displacement of the intraarticular split. If this is less than 2 mm, the fracture can be treated nonoperatively with 6 weeks in a below-elbow moulded cast.

A 17-year-old male attends the ED. He tripped over whilst jogging in the park and landed on the palm of his left hand. His hand is swollen and very painful. There is no significant past medical history. On examination, there is tenderness over the ulnar aspect of the left wrist. Grip strength is reduced. Distal pulses are present and sensory and motor function is preserved. The injury is closed.

AP and lateral X-rays of the left wrist are requested to assess for a fracture.

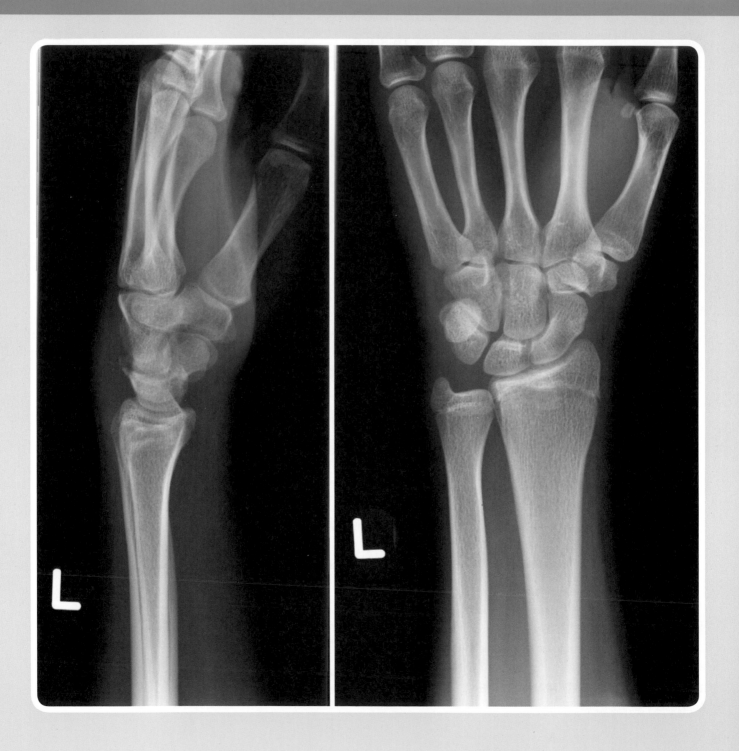

TECHNICAL INFORMATION

Patient ID: Anonymous.
Area: Left wrist.
Projection: AP and lateral.
Technical adequacy:

- Adequate coverage.
- Adequate exposure.
- The patient is not rotated.

● FRACTURE DETAILS

There is a small bony fragment dorsal to the proximal carpal row that is consistent with a triquetral fracture.

The fracture is transverse, simple and extraarticular.

There is no displacement.

There is no angulation.

There is no rotation.

There is no shortening.

● JOINTS

There is no subluxation or dislocation.

There are no loose bodies.

There is no effusion or lipohaemarthrosis.

There are no arthritic changes.

● SOFT TISSUES

There is soft tissue swelling present.

There is no surgical emphysema.

● BACKGROUND BONE

The background bone is normal.

● BONE LESIONS

There is no bone lesion present.

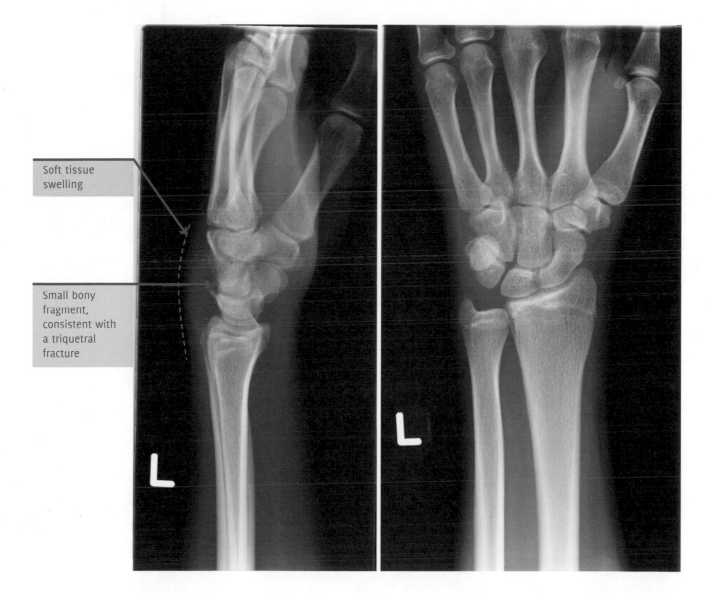

Soft tissue swelling

Small bony fragment, consistent with a triquetral fracture

SUMMARY AND DIFFERENTIAL

The lateral X-ray demonstrates a left triquetral fracture.

INVESTIGATIONS AND MANAGEMENT

Analgesia should be provided.

A Velcro wrist splint should be applied and worn the majority of the time for around 4–6 weeks. As pain subsides, the patient can begin gentle range of movement exercises. If swelling, pain and stiffness are an issue, then early referral to hand therapy is advised.

A 20-year-old student presents to the ED, having fallen whilst ice skating. She reports landing on her left forearm. There is no significant past medical history. On examination, there is an obvious deformity with swelling and bruising of the left forearm. Distal pulses are present and sensory and motor function is preserved. The injury is closed.

AP and lateral X-rays of the left forearm inclusive of the elbow and wrist are requested to assess for a fracture.

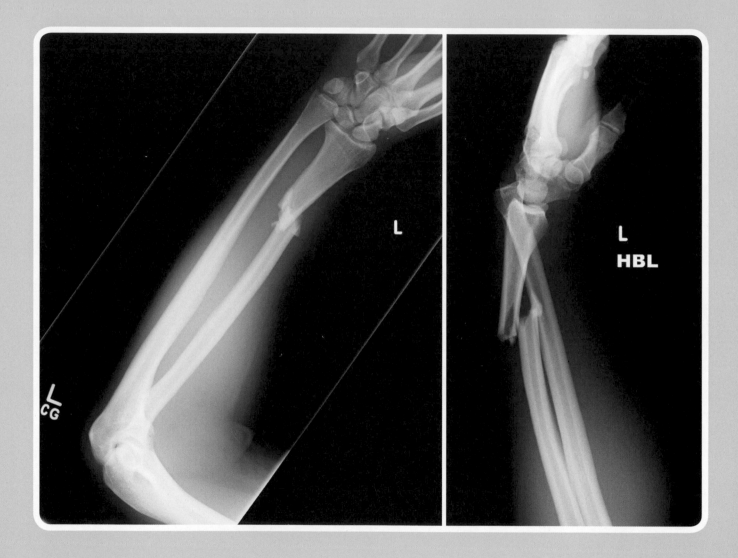

TECHNICAL INFORMATION

Patient ID: Anonymous.
Area: Left forearm.
Projection: AP and lateral.
Technical adequacy:

- Adequate coverage on the AP view.
- Inadequate coverage on the lateral view as it does not include the elbow joint.
- Adequate exposure.
- The patient is not rotated.

● FRACTURE DETAILS

There is a diaphyseal fracture of the distal third of the radius.

The fracture is oblique, comminuted and extraarticular.

There is dorsal (posterior) and medial (towards the ulnar) displacement of the distal fracture fragment.

There is volar angulation of approximately 30 degrees.

There is no rotation.

There is shortening.

● JOINTS

There is a dislocation of the distal radioulnar joint.

The elbow joint appears congruent, although this has not been fully assessed.

There are no loose bodies.

There is no effusion or lipohaemarthrosis visible.

There are no arthritic changes.

● SOFT TISSUES

There is no soft tissue swelling.

There is no surgical emphysema.

● BACKGROUND BONE

The background bone is normal.

● BONE LESIONS

There is no bone lesion present.

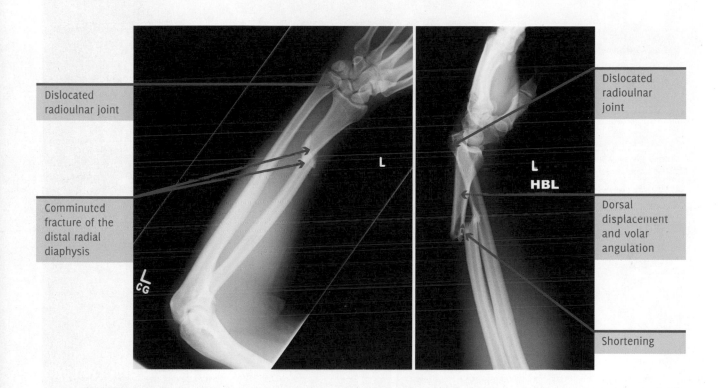

Dislocated radioulnar joint

Comminuted fracture of the distal radial diaphysis

Dislocated radioulnar joint

Dorsal displacement and volar angulation

Shortening

SUMMARY AND DIFFERENTIAL

These X-rays demonstrate a displaced fracture of the distal third of the radial diaphysis. There is an associated dislocation of the radioulnar joint, consistent with a Galeazzi fracture-dislocation.

INVESTIGATIONS AND MANAGEMENT

A lateral X-ray of the elbow is required.

Appropriate analgesia should be provided.

The patient should undergo attempted reduction in ED under sedation with orthopaedics present. A moulded back slab should be applied, and an X-ray taken to check its position. Galeazzi fracture-dislocations require surgery and therefore need early referral to orthopaedics.

A 4-year-old boy fell whilst on a trampoline, injuring his right arm. He has been brought into the ED by his parents. There is no significant past medical history. On examination, there is an obvious deformity and swelling around the forearm. Distal pulses are present and sensory and motor function is preserved. The injury is closed.

AP and lateral X-rays of the right forearm are requested to assess for a fracture.

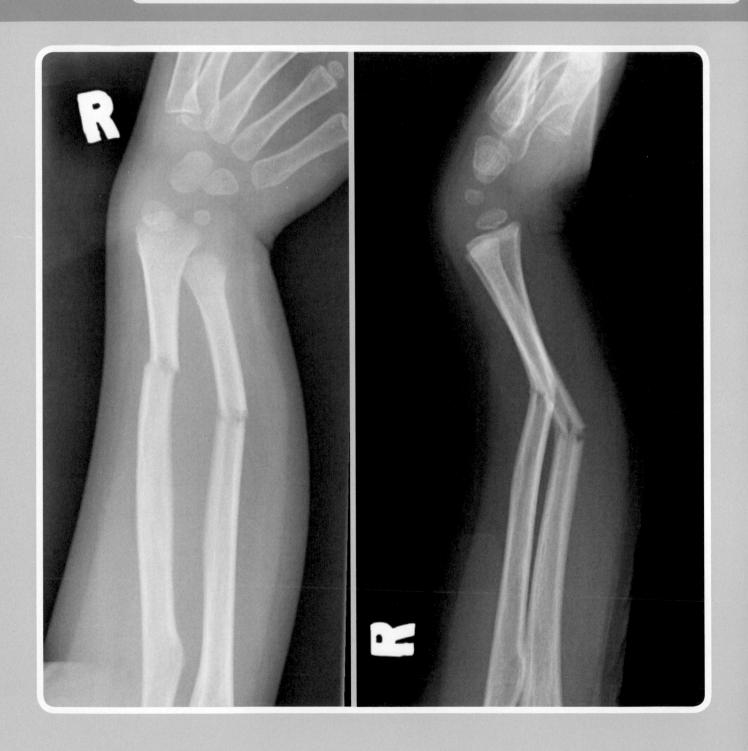

TECHNICAL INFORMATION

Patient ID: Anonymous.
Area: Right forearm.
Projection: AP and lateral.
Technical adequacy:

- Inadequate coverage – the elbow is not included on either view.
- Adequate exposure.
- The patient is not rotated.

● FRACTURE DETAILS

There is a diaphysis fracture involving the distal third of the radius.

The fracture is transverse, simple and extraarticular.

There is no displacement.

There is marked dorsal angulation of approximately 30 degrees.

There is no rotation.

There is no shortening.

There is a diaphyseal fracture involving the distal third of the ulnar.

The fracture is transverse, simple and extraarticular.

There is no displacement.

There is marked dorsal angulation of approximately 45 degrees and approximately 15 degrees of radial angulation.

There is no rotation.

There is no shortening.

● JOINTS

There is no subluxation or dislocation.

There are no loose bodies.

There is no effusion or lipohaemarthrosis.

There are no arthritic changes.

● SOFT TISSUES

There is no soft tissue swelling.

There is no surgical emphysema.

● BACKGROUND BONE

The background bone is normal.

● BONE LESIONS

There is no bone lesion present.

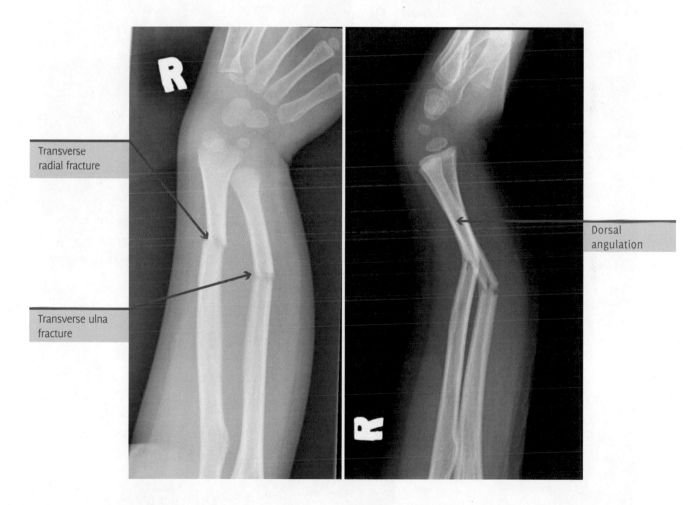

Transverse radial fracture

Transverse ulna fracture

Dorsal angulation

SUMMARY AND DIFFERENTIAL

These X-rays demonstrate a dorsally angulated fracture of the distal third of both the radius and ulna.

INVESTIGATIONS AND MANAGEMENT

Appropriate analgesia should be provided.

Repeat X-rays, adequately including the elbow, should be performed.

The patient should undergo reduction in the ED by orthopaedics under sedation. This can often be achieved with a mixture of intranasal diamorphine and Entonox. A moulded full cast should be applied, and an X-ray taken to check position. If the position is satisfactory, then a follow-up X-ray at 1 week is required to ensure there is no redisplacement. The parents should be advised to elevate the limb and watch for swelling.

If the reduction is inadequate, the orthopaedic surgeon may consider further manipulation in theatre +/− flexible intramedullary nails.

A 10-year-old boy was playing rugby at school when he was tackled and fell to the ground. The other player landed on top of him. Subsequently, he felt a 'snap' and presents to the ED with a visibly deformed arm. There is no significant past medical history. On examination, the arm is visibly deformed. There is swelling and tenderness around the mid-forearm. Distal pulses are present. Altered sensation is reported in all fingers but motor function is preserved. The injury is closed.

AP and lateral X-rays of the left forearm are requested to assess for a fracture.

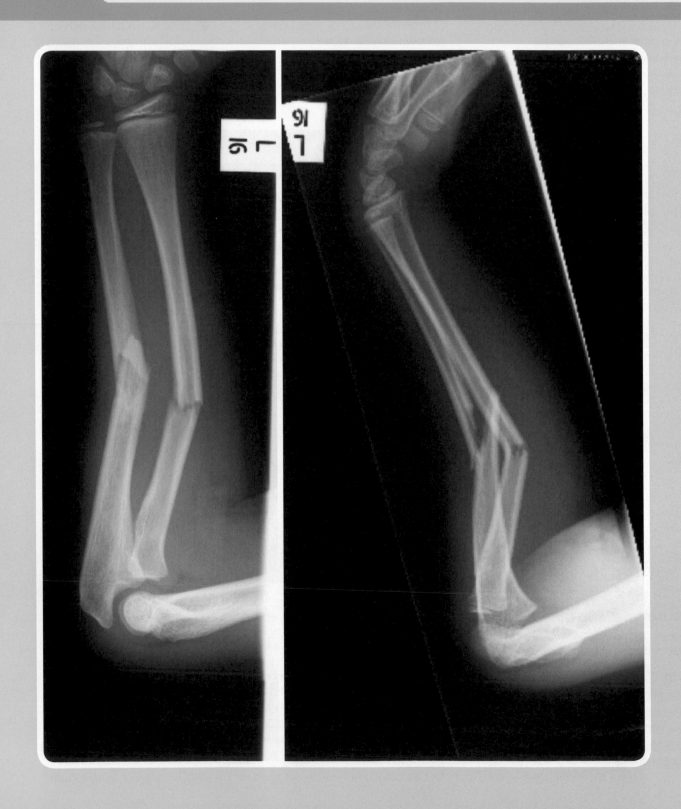

TECHNICAL INFORMATION

Patient ID: Anonymous.
Area: Left radius and ulna.
Projection: AP and lateral.
Technical adequacy:

- Adequate coverage.
- Adequate exposure.
- The patient is not rotated.

● FRACTURE DETAILS

There is a fracture involving the middle third of the radius (diaphysis).

The fracture is transverse, simple and extraarticular.

There is no displacement.

Dorsal and medial (towards the ulna) angulation is present.

There is no rotation.

There is no shortening.

There is a similar fracture involving the middle third of the ulna (diaphysis).

The fracture is oblique, simple and extraarticular.

There is no displacement.

Dorsal and medial (towards the ulna) angulation is present.

There is no rotation.

There is no shortening.

● JOINTS

There is no subluxation or dislocation of the distal radioulnar joint or elbow joint.

There are no loose bodies.

There is no effusion or lipohaemarthrosis.

There are no arthritic changes.

● SOFT TISSUES

Soft tissue swelling is noted around the proximal forearm.

There is no surgical emphysema.

● BACKGROUND BONE

The background bone is normal.

● BONE LESIONS

There is no bone lesion present.

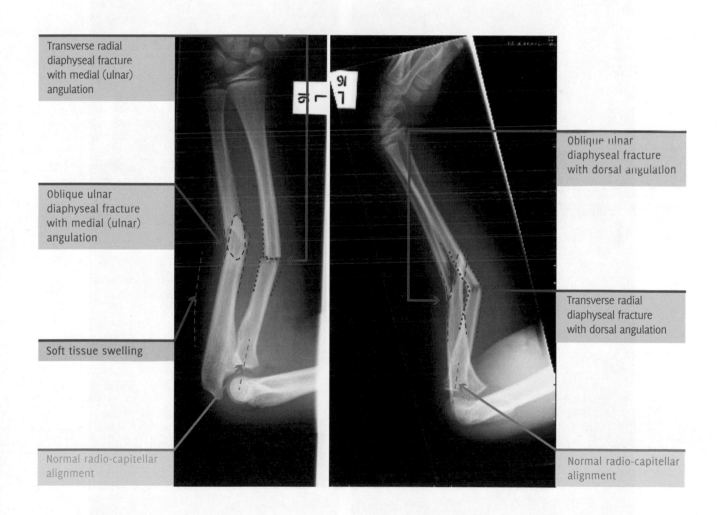

Transverse radial diaphyseal fracture with medial (ulnar) angulation

Oblique ulnar diaphyseal fracture with medial (ulnar) angulation

Soft tissue swelling

Normal radio-capitellar alignment

Oblique ulnar diaphyseal fracture with dorsal angulation

Transverse radial diaphyseal fracture with dorsal angulation

Normal radio-capitellar alignment

SUMMARY AND DIFFERENTIAL

These X-rays demonstrate displaced fractures of the mid-radial and mid-ulnar diaphysis.

INVESTIGATIONS AND MANAGEMENT

Appropriate analgesia should be provided.

The arm should be immobilized in an above-elbow back slab.

A referral should be made to an orthopaedic surgeon for operative fixation, which may be with ORIF or intramedullary flexible titanium nails.

A 7-year-old boy presents to ED after he fell from the top of a climbing frame onto an outstretched right hand. There is no significant past medical history. On examination, there is a deformed forearm with swelling around the elbow. The patient is tender over the anterior aspect of the elbow and mid-forearm. Distal pulses are present and motor and sensory function is preserved. The injury is closed.

AP and lateral X-rays of the right forearm including the elbow are requested to assess for a fracture.

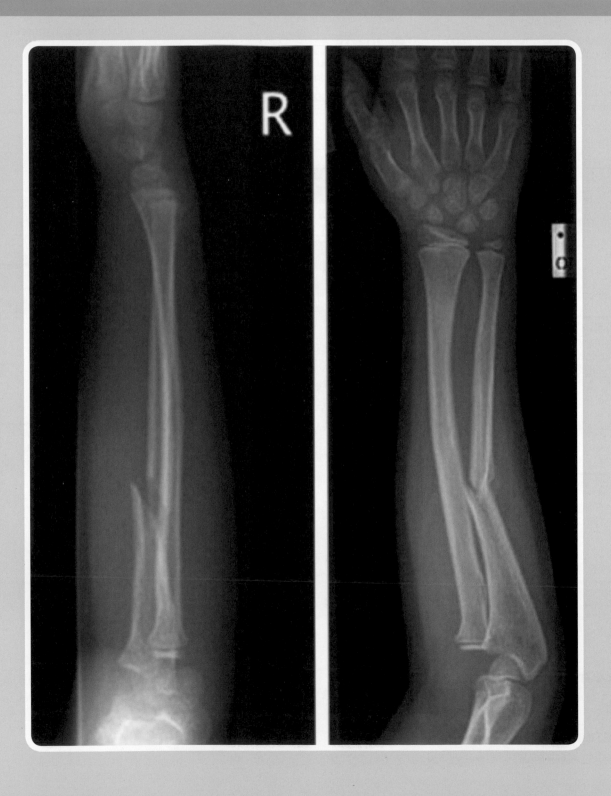

TECHNICAL INFORMATION

Patient ID: Anonymous.
Area: Right forearm including the elbow.
Projection: AP and lateral.
Technical adequacy:

- Adequate coverage.
- Adequate exposure.
- The patient is not rotated.

● FRACTURE DETAILS

There is a fracture involving the proximal third of the right ulna (diaphysis).

The fracture is oblique, simple and extraarticular.

There is dorsal displacement of approximately 5 mm.

There is medial (ulnar) angulation of approximately 30 degrees.

There is no rotation.

There is no shortening.

● JOINTS

There is an anterior dislocation of the radial head.

There are no loose bodies.

There is no effusion or lipohaemarthrosis.

There are no arthritic changes.

● SOFT TISSUES

There is soft tissue swelling present on the radial border of the forearm.

There is no surgical emphysema,

● BACKGROUND BONE

The background bone is normal.

● BONE LESIONS

There is no bone lesion present.

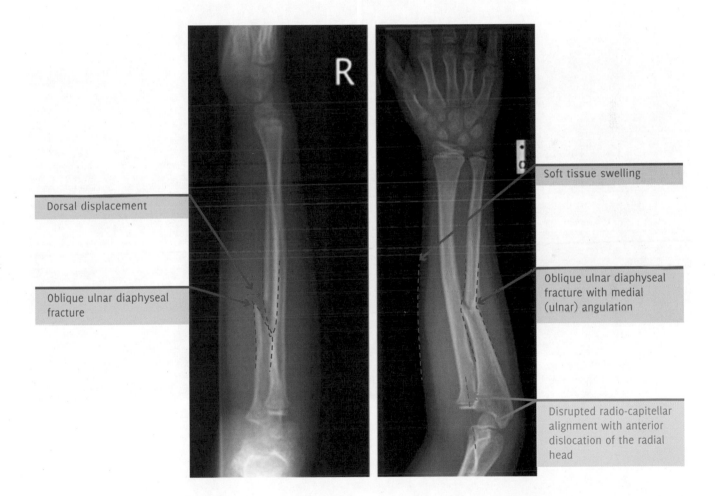

Soft tissue swelling

Dorsal displacement

Oblique ulnar diaphyseal fracture

Oblique ulnar diaphyseal fracture with medial (ulnar) angulation

Disrupted radio-capitellar alignment with anterior dislocation of the radial head

SUMMARY AND DIFFERENTIAL

These X-rays demonstrate an angulated and displaced ulnar diaphyseal fracture. There is associated dislocation of the radial head. The injury pattern is consistent with a Monteggia fracture-dislocation.

INVESTIGATIONS AND MANAGEMENT

Appropriate analgesia should be provided.

An above-elbow back slab should be applied. The patient should be referred to orthopaedics. The ulna needs anatomical reduction to allow the radial head dislocation to reduce and so this fracture may well require ORIF.

A 78-year-old woman presents to the ED having fallen down five stairs. She thinks she landed on a flexed right arm. She has a past medical history of atrial fibrillation and hypertension. On arrival in the ED, a full ATLS assessment is performed identifying no immediate life- or limb-threatening injuries. On examination during the secondary survey, there is tenderness, swelling and bruising over the right elbow. The patient has reduced elbow extension but can manage a small amount of flexion with pain. Distal pulses are present and sensory and motor function is preserved. The injury is closed.

AP and lateral X-rays of the right elbow are requested to assess for fracture.

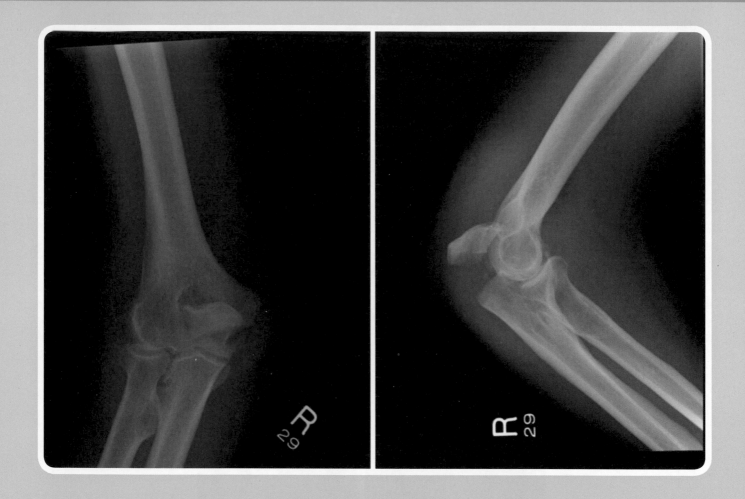

TECHNICAL INFORMATION

Patient ID: Anonymous.
Area: Right elbow.
Projection: AP and lateral.
Technical adequacy:

- Adequate coverage.
- Adequate exposure.
- The patient is not rotated.

● FRACTURE DETAILS

There is a fracture of the olecranon.

The fracture is transverse, simple and intraarticular.

There is marked posterior displacement.

There is angulation.

There is no rotation.

There is no shortening.

There is also a bony fragment adjacent to the site of the medial epicondyle. This fragment appears well corticated and may represent a previous fracture, but this may also represent another acute fracture as a differential diagnosis.

● JOINTS

There is no subluxation or dislocation. In particular, the radio-capitellar line is normal.

There are no loose bodies.

There is elevation of the anterior fat pad, in keeping with a joint effusion.

There are degenerative changes at the radio-capitellar compartment, with osteophyte formation.

● SOFT TISSUES

There is significant soft tissue swelling.

There is no surgical emphysema.

● BACKGROUND BONE

The background bone is normal.

● BONE LESIONS

There is no bone lesion present.

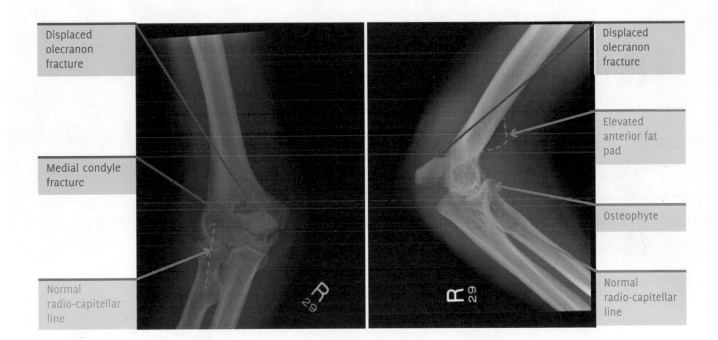

Displaced olecranon fracture

Medial condyle fracture

Normal radio-capitellar line

Displaced olecranon fracture

Elevated anterior fat pad

Osteophyte

Normal radio-capitellar line

SUMMARY AND DIFFERENTIAL

Both X-rays demonstrate a displaced intraarticular olecranon fracture. There may be an associated fracture of the medial condyle of the humerus, but this more likely represents an old injury.

INVESTIGATIONS AND MANAGEMENT

Appropriate analgesia should be provided.

The patient can be managed initially in either a broad arm sling or above-elbow back slab depending on pain.

A referral should be made to an orthopaedic surgeon to consider ORIF with tension band wire fixation of the olecranon, followed by early range of movement exercises at 2 weeks after surgery.

A 60-year-old judo instructor fell onto his outstretched arm whilst demonstrating a grappling technique. Bystanders noted a deformity to the arm and the patient was in significant pain, so an ambulance was called. There is no significant past medical history. On examination, there is an obviously deformed right elbow. Distal pulses are present but there is paraesthesia in the median nerve distribution. Sensory and motor function is otherwise preserved. The injury is closed.

AP and lateral X-rays of the right elbow are requested to assess for fracture.

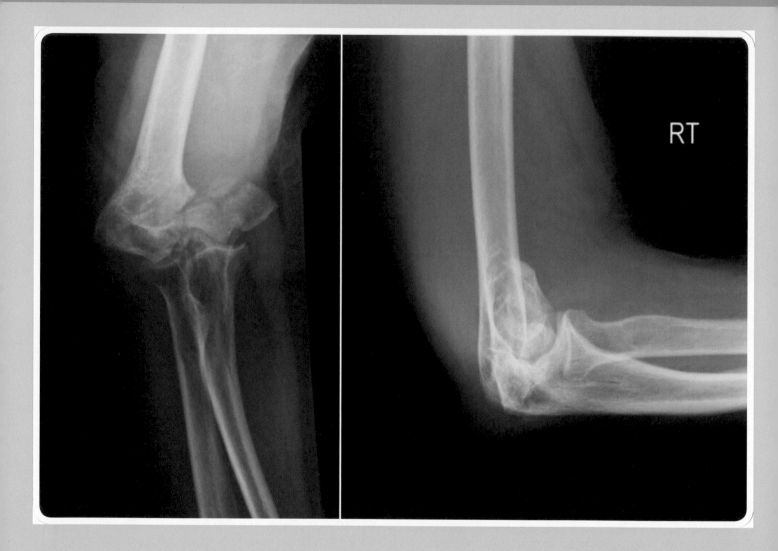

TECHNICAL INFORMATION

Patient ID: Anonymous.
Area: Right elbow.
Projection: AP and lateral.
Technical adequacy:

- Adequate coverage.
- Adequate exposure.
- The patient is not rotated.

● FRACTURE DETAILS

There is a fracture involving the condyles of the distal humerus.

The exact fracture pattern is difficult to assess but there appears to be a T-shaped, comminuted and intraarticular fracture.

There is marked medial and anterior displacement of the distal fracture fragments.

There is angulation.

There is rotation.

There is marked shortening present.

● JOINTS

Congruency of the joint is difficult to assess, but there is a subluxation of the elbow joint on the AP. There is no dislocation visible.

There are fracture fragments and loose bodies within the joint space.

There is no effusion or lipohaemarthrosis visible.

There are no arthritic changes.

● SOFT TISSUES

There is significant tissue swelling.

There is no surgical emphysema.

● BACKGROUND BONE

The background bone is normal.

● BONE LESIONS

There is no bone lesion present.

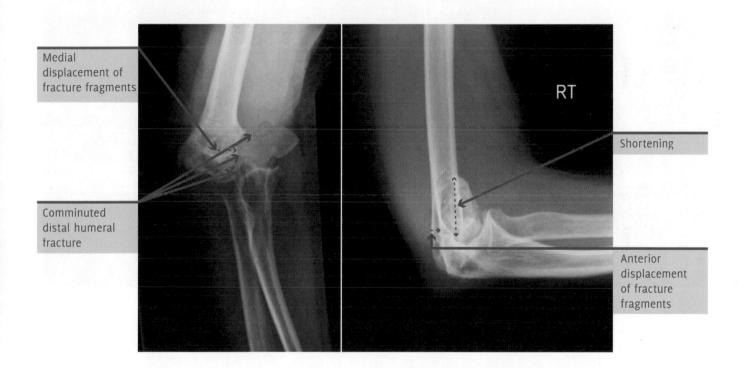

Medial displacement of fracture fragments

Comminuted distal humeral fracture

RT

Shortening

Anterior displacement of fracture fragments

SUMMARY AND DIFFERENTIAL

Both X-rays demonstrate a comminuted intraarticular fracture of the right distal humerus, with an associated subluxation of the elbow joint.

INVESTIGATIONS AND MANAGEMENT

Appropriate analgesia should be provided.

An above-elbow back slab should be applied, and an X-ray taken to check positioning. Repeat clinical assessment should be performed to assess for distal pulses and motor and sensory function.

A CT scan of the elbow should be requested to further assess the fracture.

An urgent referral should be made to an orthopaedic surgeon who may consider ORIF. If the fracture is too severe or the articular fragments are too comminuted, then the surgeon may also consider total elbow replacement.

A 24-year-old woman fell onto her outstretched right hand whilst intoxicated at a nightclub. She presents to the ED the following morning. There is no significant past medical history. On examination, there is a limited range of movement due to pain. There is no obvious bruising. However, tenderness over the radial head is present. The injury is closed and neurovascularly intact.

AP and lateral X-rays of the right elbow are requested to assess for fracture.

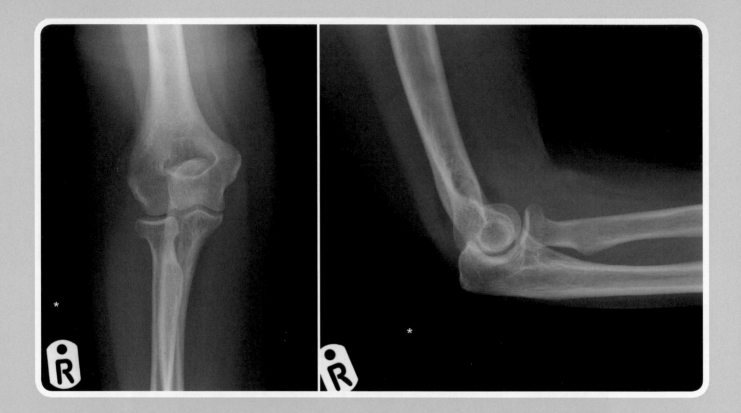

TECHNICAL INFORMATION

Patient ID: Anonymous.
Area: Right elbow.
Projection: AP and lateral.
Technical adequacy:

- Adequate coverage.
- Adequate exposure.
- The patient is not rotated.

● FRACTURE DETAILS

There is a displaced fracture of the radial neck.

The fracture is transverse, simple and intraarticular although not involving the articular surface of the radial head.

There is minimal displacement.

There is no angulation.

There is no rotation.

There is no shortening.

● JOINTS

There is no subluxation or dislocation. In particular, the radio-capitellar line is normal.

There are no loose bodies.

There are anterior and posterior fat pad signs, consistent with an effusion.

There are no arthritic changes.

● SOFT TISSUES

There is no soft tissue swelling.

There is no surgical emphysema.

● BACKGROUND BONE

The background bone is normal.

● BONE LESIONS

There is no bone lesion present.

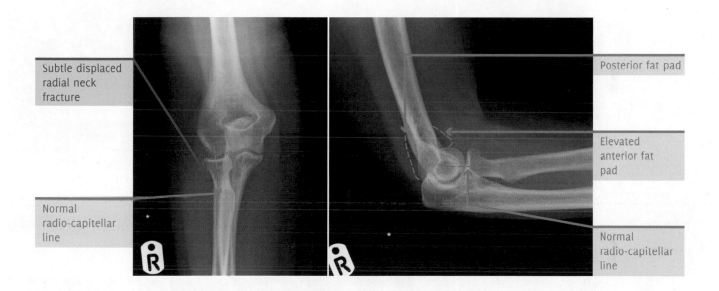

Subtle displaced radial neck fracture

Normal radio-capitellar line

Posterior fat pad

Elevated anterior fat pad

Normal radio-capitellar line

SUMMARY AND DIFFERENTIAL

Both X-rays demonstrate an undisplaced radial neck fracture with an associated elbow joint effusion.

INVESTIGATIONS AND MANAGEMENT

Appropriate analgesia should be provided.

A broad arm sling should be fitted.

The patient can begin early range of movement exercises as pain allows and should be referred to a fracture clinic.

A 6-year-old boy fell on his outstretched arm whilst playing football. He is refusing to move his elbow as he is complaining of elbow pain. There is no significant past medical history. On examination, there is a swollen right elbow, particularly over the lateral aspect. The pain is exacerbated by movement of the elbow and is worst on supination and pronation. Distal pulses are present and sensory and motor function is preserved. The injury is closed.

AP and lateral X-rays of the right elbow are requested to assess for a fracture.

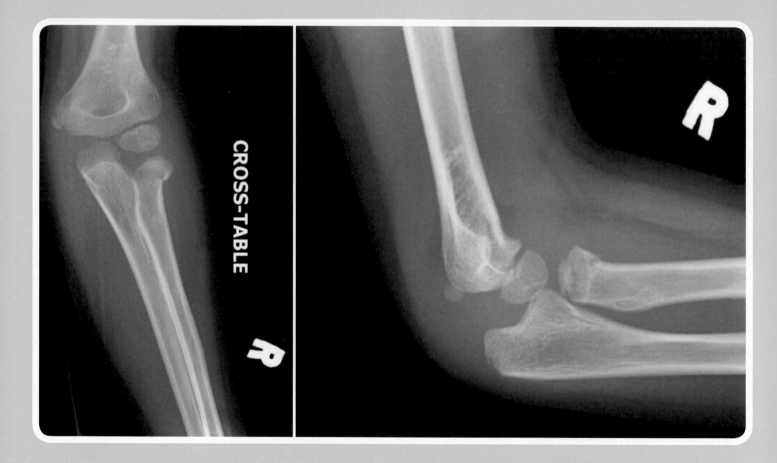

CROSS-TABLE

TECHNICAL INFORMATION

Patient ID: Anonymous.
Area: Right elbow.
Projection: AP and lateral.
Technical adequacy:

- Adequate coverage.
- Adequate exposure.
- The patient is not rotated.

● FRACTURE DETAILS

There is a fracture involving the metaphysis of the radial neck, extending to the physis.

The fracture is oblique, simple and extraarticular.

There is no translational displacement.

There is ~40 degrees of angulation present.

There is no rotation.

There is no shortening.

● JOINTS

There is no subluxation or dislocation of the elbow joint.

There are no loose bodies.

There are anterior and posterior fat pad signs, indicating an elbow joint effusion.

There are no arthritic changes.

● SOFT TISSUES

There is no soft tissue swelling visible.

There is no surgical emphysema.

● BACKGROUND BONE

The background bone is normal.

● BONE LESIONS

There is no bone lesion present.

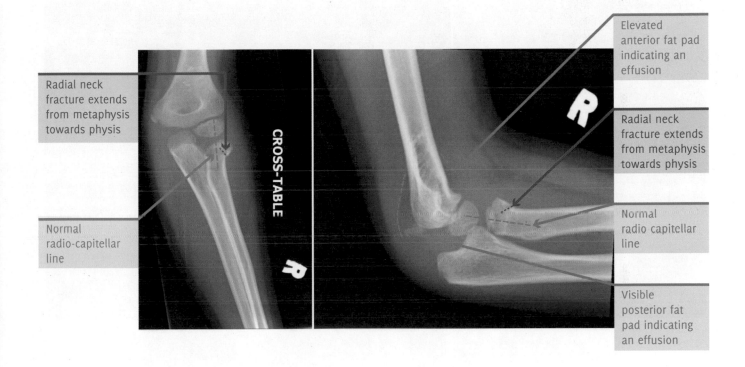

Radial neck fracture extends from metaphysis towards physis

Normal radio-capitellar line

CROSS-TABLE

Elevated anterior fat pad indicating an effusion

Radial neck fracture extends from metaphysis towards physis

Normal radio capitellar line

Visible posterior fat pad indicating an effusion

SUMMARY AND DIFFERENTIAL

These X-rays demonstrate a significantly angulated radial neck fracture. The fracture involves the physis and metaphysis, consistent with a Salter-Harris Type 2 fracture.

INVESTIGATIONS AND MANAGEMENT

Appropriate analgesia should be provided.

The arm should be immobilized in an above-elbow back slab. The patient should be referred to orthopaedics for consideration of MUA in theatre.

A 5-year-old girl was on a trampoline with her older brother. Her father saw her fall off the trampoline and land on an extended right arm. She presents with obvious elbow deformity and swelling. There is no significant past medical history. On examination, there is swelling and tenderness around the elbow. Minimal movement exacerbates the pain. Distal pulses are present and sensory and motor function is preserved. The injury is closed.

AP and lateral X-rays of the right elbow are requested to assess for a fracture.

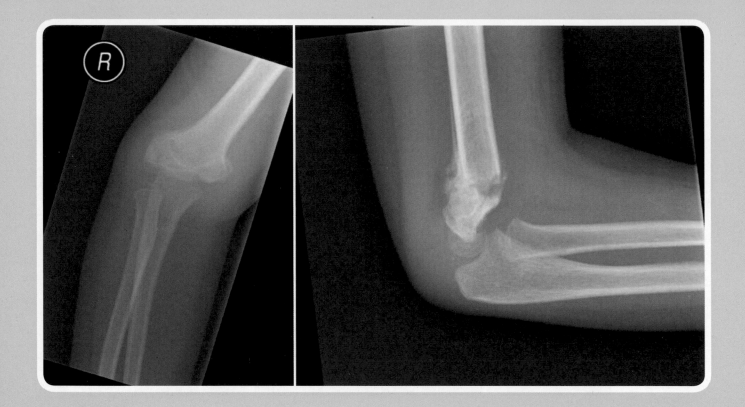

TECHNICAL INFORMATION

Patient ID: Anonymous.
Area: Right elbow.
Projection: AP and lateral.
Technical adequacy:

- Adequate coverage.
- Adequate exposure.
- The patient is not rotated.

● FRACTURE DETAILS

There is a fracture involving the supracondylar region of the humerus.

The fracture is transverse, simple and extraarticular.

There is no displacement.

There is posterior angulation present.

There is no rotation.

There is no shortening.

● JOINTS

There is no subluxation or dislocation.

There are no loose bodies.

There is elbow joint effusion present.

There are no arthritic changes.

● SOFT TISSUES

There is soft tissue swelling around the elbow.

There is no surgical emphysema.

● BACKGROUND BONE

The background bone is normal.

● BONE LESIONS

There is no bone lesion present.

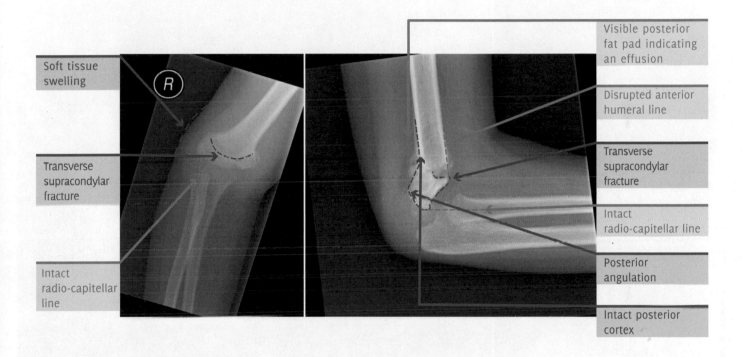

Soft tissue swelling

Transverse supracondylar fracture

Intact radio-capitellar line

Visible posterior fat pad indicating an effusion

Disrupted anterior humeral line

Transverse supracondylar fracture

Intact radio-capitellar line

Posterior angulation

Intact posterior cortex

SUMMARY AND DIFFERENTIAL

Both X-rays demonstrate a posteriorly angulated supracondylar fracture. The posterior cortex of the distal humerus appears intact. This represents a Gartland Type 2 fracture.

INVESTIGATIONS AND MANAGEMENT

Advice regarding analgesia should be provided.

A temporary above-elbow back slab should be placed in the resting position of the elbow with neurovascular status checked afterwards, ensuring pulses, CRT and individual nerve function are assessed and results documented.

A referral should be made to orthopaedics who will likely proceed with operative fixation with MUA and K wires, followed by a period of immobilization in an above-elbow cast.

A 33-year-old right-hand-dominant estate agent has injured his left elbow after being tackled whilst playing rugby. He has been driven to the ED by a teammate. There is no significant past medical history. On examination, the elbow is swollen and bruised with limited range of movement secondary to pain. Distal pulses are present and sensory and motor function is preserved. Specifically, the radial nerve is intact. The injury is closed.

AP and lateral X-rays of the left humerus are requested to assess for a fracture.

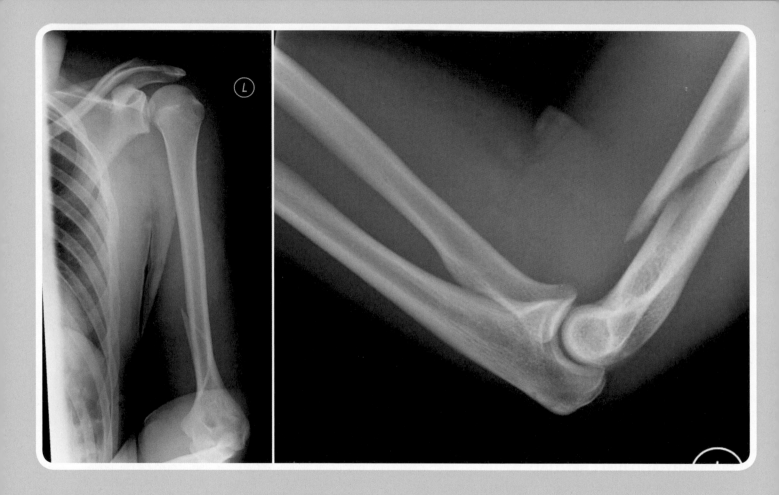

TECHNICAL INFORMATION

Patient ID: Anonymous.
Area: Left distal humerus.
Projection: AP mortise and lateral.
Technical adequacy:

- Inadequate coverage – the AP view has satisfactory coverage. However, the lateral view does not include the entire humerus or the glenohumeral joint.
- Adequate exposure.
- The patient is not rotated.

● FRACTURE DETAILS

There is a fracture involving the distal humerus.

The fracture is spiral, simple and extraarticular.

There is minimal posterior displacement and minimal lateral angulation.

There is rotation.

There is shortening.

● JOINTS

There is no subluxation or dislocation.

There are no loose bodies.

There is no effusion or lipohaemarthrosis.

There are no arthritic changes.

● SOFT TISSUES

There is no soft tissue swelling.

There is no surgical emphysema.

● BACKGROUND BONE

The background bone is normal.

● BONE LESIONS

There is no bone lesion present.

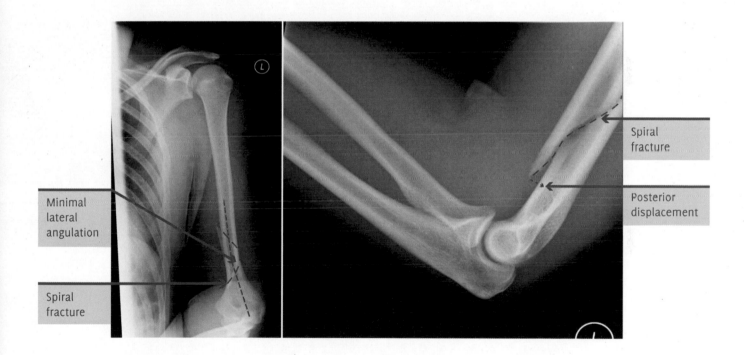

Minimal lateral angulation

Spiral fracture

Spiral fracture

Posterior displacement

SUMMARY AND DIFFERENTIAL

These X-rays demonstrate a minimally displaced spiral fracture of the distal humerus.

INVESTIGATIONS AND MANAGEMENT

Appropriate analgesia should be provided.

The lateral X-ray should be repeated to ensure adequate coverage. The patient should be given a broad arm sling and following this, repeat assessment of distal pulses and sensory and motor function should be performed. This fracture is very close to the path of the radial nerve, which can become trapped in the fracture site leading to a palsy.

The patient should be referred to orthopaedics for consideration of ORIF.

SHOULDER GIRDLE

A 72-year-old retired teacher attends the ED after tripping over a curb near his golf club. He describes falling onto his left shoulder. He also reports that his shoulder became instantly painful, and he has since been unable to move it. There is no significant past medical history. On examination, there is swelling and bruising around the left shoulder. There is tenderness on palpation. All movements of the shoulder are limited because of pain. Distal pulses are present and sensory and motor function is preserved including the axillary nerve. The injury is closed.

AP and scapula-Y view X-rays of the left shoulder are requested to assess for a fracture or dislocation.

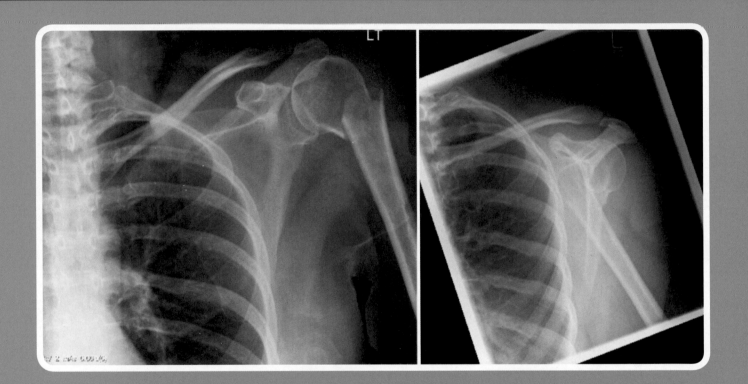

TECHNICAL INFORMATION

Patient ID: Anonymous.
Area: Left shoulder.
Projection: AP and scapula-Y.
Technical adequacy:

- Adequate coverage.
- Adequate exposure.
- The patient is not rotated.

● FRACTURE DETAILS

There is a fracture involving the proximal humerus at the surgical neck.

The fracture is transverse, simple and extraarticular.

There is marked anterior displacement of the distal fragment (humeral neck and shaft).

There is slight medial angulation.

There is no rotation.

There is shortening of approximately 2 mm.

● JOINTS

There is no subluxation or dislocation of the glenohumeral or acromioclavicular joints.

There are no loose bodies.

There is no effusion or lipohaemarthrosis.

There are no arthritic changes.

● SOFT TISSUES

There is no soft tissue swelling.

There is no surgical emphysema.

The imaged left lung is clear.

● BACKGROUND BONE

The background bone is normal.

● BONE LESIONS

There is no bone lesion present.

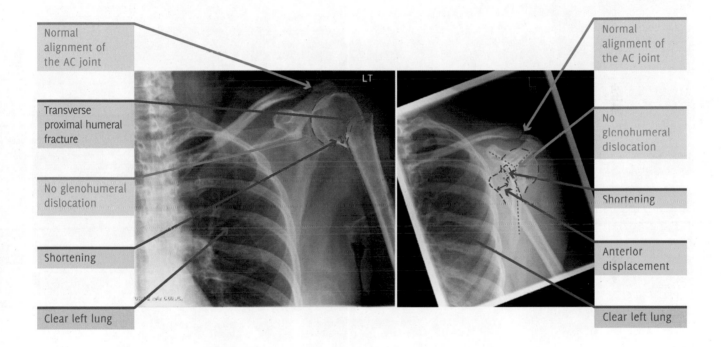

Normal alignment of the AC joint

Transverse proximal humeral fracture

No glenohumeral dislocation

Shortening

Clear left lung

Normal alignment of the AC joint

No glenohumeral dislocation

Shortening

Anterior displacement

Clear left lung

SUMMARY AND DIFFERENTIAL

Both X-rays demonstrate a transverse left proximal humeral fracture with significant anterior displacement. The fracture is simple and extraarticular and there is no glenohumeral joint dislocation.

INVESTIGATIONS AND MANAGEMENT

Advice regarding analgesia should be provided.

A collar and cuff should be fitted for immobilization. The patient should be referred to fracture clinic for ongoing management. Options for management include ORIF or nonoperative treatment.

A 32-year-old female has been brought to the ED by ambulance after having a tonic-clonic seizure. She is known to suffer from epilepsy and has been struggling to take her antiepileptic medication because of recent vomiting and diarrhoea. On recovery from her seizure, she complains of pain in her right shoulder. There is no significant past medical history other than epilepsy. The patient does state this has happened before and that she required surgical stabilization. On examination, there is loss of the right shoulder contour, with a prominent coracoid and posterior shoulder position. There is pain on moving the shoulder in any direction. Distal pulses are present and sensation is preserved, including the axillary nerve. A complete motor assessment is not possible because of pain. The injury is closed.

AP and oblique X-rays of the right shoulder joint are requested to assess for fracture or dislocation.

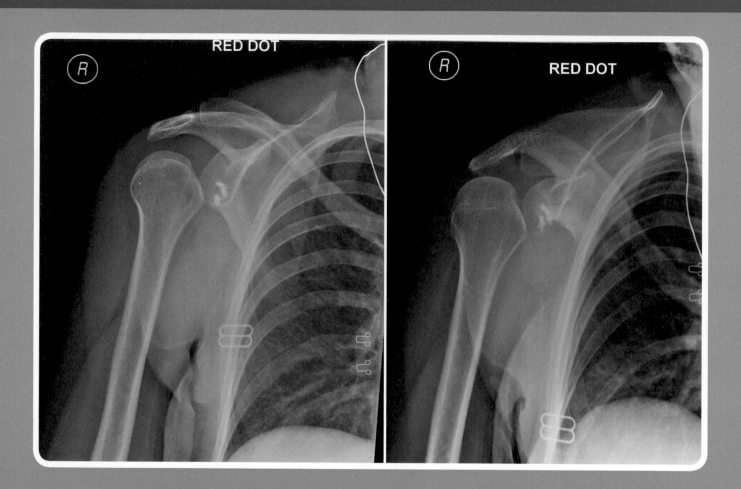

TECHNICAL INFORMATION

Patient ID: Anonymous.
Area: Right shoulder.
Projection: AP and apical oblique.
Technical adequacy:

- Adequate coverage.
- Adequate exposure.
- The patient is not rotated.

● FRACTURE DETAILS

There is no fracture.

● JOINTS

There is a posterior dislocation of the right humeral head – note positive 'lightbulb' sign.

There are no loose bodies.

There is no effusion or lipohaemarthrosis.

There are no arthritic changes.

● SOFT TISSUES

There is no soft tissue swelling.

There is no surgical emphysema.

The imaged right lung is clear.

● BACKGROUND BONE

There are several implants in the glenoid, which represent bone anchors. This suggests the patient has previously had a shoulder stabilization procedure.

● BONE LESIONS

There is no bone lesion present.

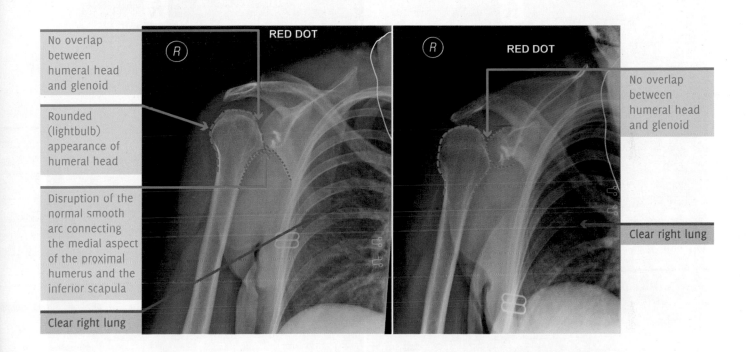

SUMMARY AND DIFFERENTIAL

Both X-rays demonstrate a right posterior shoulder dislocation with evidence of previous shoulder stabilization surgery.

INVESTIGATIONS AND MANAGEMENT

Advice regarding analgesia should be provided.

The dislocation should be reduced under sedation. A broad arm sling should be provided with a block to prevent internal rotation. The patient should be referred to fracture clinic and for urgent physiotherapy with advice to avoid adduction and internal rotation.

The patient should be discussed with neurology to optimise her antiepileptic medication during the intercurrent illness.

An 84-year-old woman who lives in her own home had a witnessed mechanical fall. She has been brought to the ED by ambulance. The paramedics report that after the fall, she immediately started to complain of pain in her right shoulder and an inability to move her arm. She has a past history of hypertension and osteoporosis. On examination, there is a prominent coracoid and acromion. The humeral head is not palpable within the joint. There is substantial bruising around the shoulder. The patient is unable to move the shoulder at all. Distal pulses are present and sensory and motor function is preserved, although it is not possible to assess motor function of the axillary nerve. The injury is closed.

AP and scapula-Y view X-rays of the right shoulder are requested to assess for a fracture.

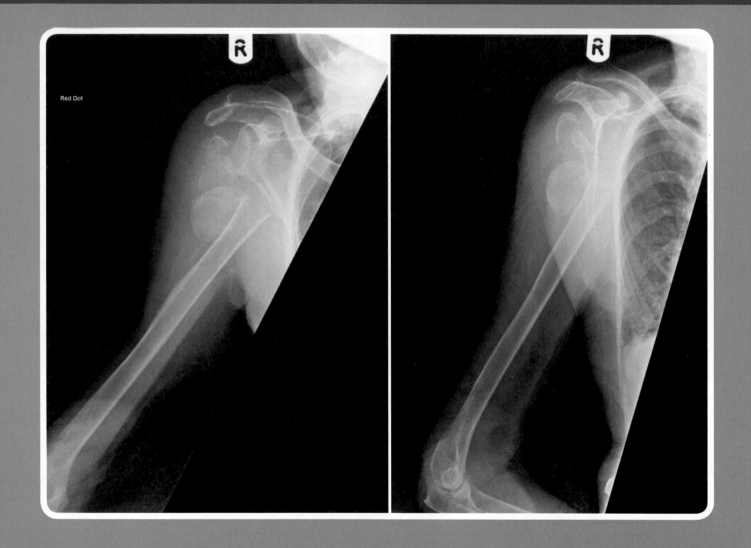

TECHNICAL INFORMATION

Patient ID: Anonymous.
Area: Right shoulder.
Projection: AP and scapula-Y.
Technical adequacy:

- Adequate coverage.
- Adequate exposure.
- The patient is not rotated.

● FRACTURE DETAILS

There is a fracture of the proximal humerus.

The fracture is transverse, comminuted and intraarticular.

There is marked anteromedial displacement of the main distal fragment.

There is no angulation.

There is no rotation.

There is marked shortening.

● JOINTS

There is a dislocation of the glenohumeral joint.

There are no loose bodies.

There is no effusion or lipohaemarthrosis.

There are no arthritic changes.

● SOFT TISSUES

There is no soft tissue swelling.

There is no surgical emphysema.

The partially imaged left lung is clear.

● BACKGROUND BONE

The background bone is osteopaenic.

● BONE LESIONS

There is no bone lesion present.

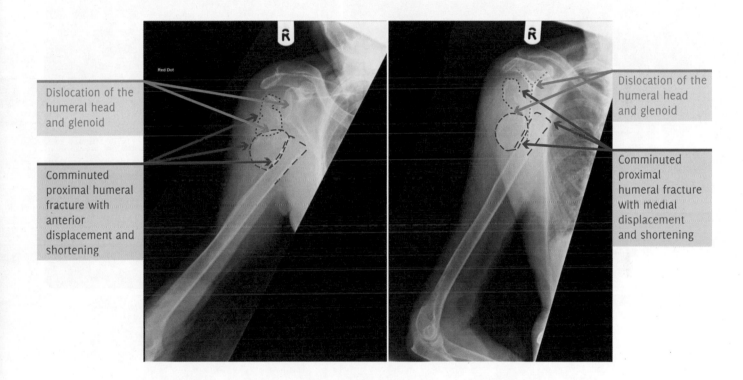

Dislocation of the humeral head and glenoid

Comminuted proximal humeral fracture with anterior displacement and shortening

Dislocation of the humeral head and glenoid

Comminuted proximal humeral fracture with medial displacement and shortening

SUMMARY AND DIFFERENTIAL

Both X-rays demonstrate a comminuted intraarticular fracture of the proximal right humerus, with associated dislocation of the right glenohumeral joint.

INVESTIGATIONS AND MANAGEMENT

Analgesia should be provided, and the arm placed in a broad arm sling. Reduction attempts will be unsuccessful and should not be attempted.

A CT scan is required to further delineate the extent of the injury and for surgical planning.

The patient should be referred to orthopaedics who will consider surgery. Options include surgical fixation or replacement of the humeral head with either a shoulder hemiarthroplasty or a reverse shoulder replacement.

A 23-year-old motorcyclist has crashed his motorbike while travelling at approximately 25 mph. He reports landing on an outstretched left arm. He now has pain in his arm but denies any other injuries. The paramedics bring him to a major trauma centre as a trauma call. After a primary and secondary survey, there is thought to be an isolated injury to the left shoulder. There is no significant past medical history. On examination, the patient is tender around the left shoulder. The acromion is prominent and is the most lateral palpable structure. All movements of the shoulder are painful. Distal pulses are present, motor function is intact, and sensation is intact in the hand. There is altered sensation over the regimental badge patch area. The injury is closed.

AP and scapula-Y view X-rays of the left shoulder are requested to assess for a fracture or dislocation.

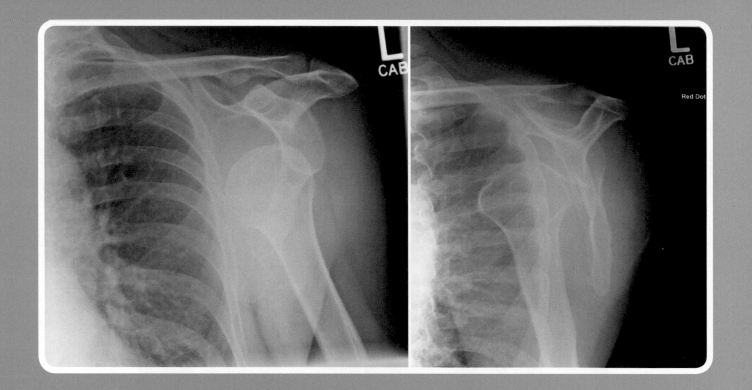

TECHNICAL INFORMATION

Patient ID: Anonymous.
Area: Left shoulder.
Projection: AP and scapula-Y.
Technical adequacy:

- Adequate coverage.
- Adequate exposure.
- The patient is not rotated.

● FRACTURE DETAILS

There is no fracture.

● JOINTS

There is an anterior dislocation of the left humeral head.

There are no loose bodies.

There is no effusion or lipohaemarthrosis.

There are no arthritic changes.

● SOFT TISSUES

There is no soft tissue swelling.

There is no surgical emphysema.

The imaged left lung is clear.

● BACKGROUND BONE

The background bone is normal.

● BONE LESIONS

There is no bone lesion present.

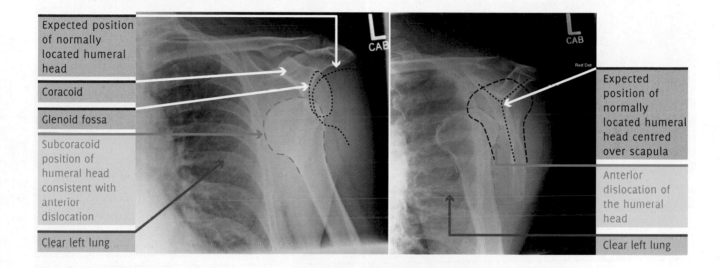

Left image labels: Expected position of normally located humeral head · Coracoid · Glenoid fossa · Subcoracoid position of humeral head consistent with anterior dislocation · Clear left lung

Right image labels: Expected position of normally located humeral head centred over scapula · Anterior dislocation of the humeral head · Clear left lung

SUMMARY AND DIFFERENTIAL

Both X-rays demonstrate an anterior dislocation of the left glenohumeral joint. No associated humeral head or glenoid fracture is visible.

INVESTIGATIONS AND MANAGEMENT

Advice regarding analgesia should be provided.

The shoulder should undergo closed reduction in ED under sedation. A check X-ray and repeat neurovascular assessment should be performed after manipulation.

The patient should be given a broad arm sling with advice to rest for 2 weeks, followed by gentle mobilization. The patient should be referred urgently to fracture clinic. The patient requires an MRI and an opinion from a shoulder surgeon. As he is under 25 years, the risk of further dislocation is high and there may be a structural injury amenable to surgery visible on the MRI.

A 69-year-old woman tripped over the edge of a rug at home. She has fallen and landed on her outstretched left arm. Since this event, she has been complaining of pain in her left arm. Her husband has brought her to the ED. There is no significant past medical history. On examination, the acromion is prominent and is the most lateral palpable structure. All movements of the shoulder are painful. Distal pulses are present and sensory and motor function is preserved including the axillary nerve. The injury is closed.

AP and apical oblique X-rays of the left shoulder are requested to assess for a fracture or dislocation.

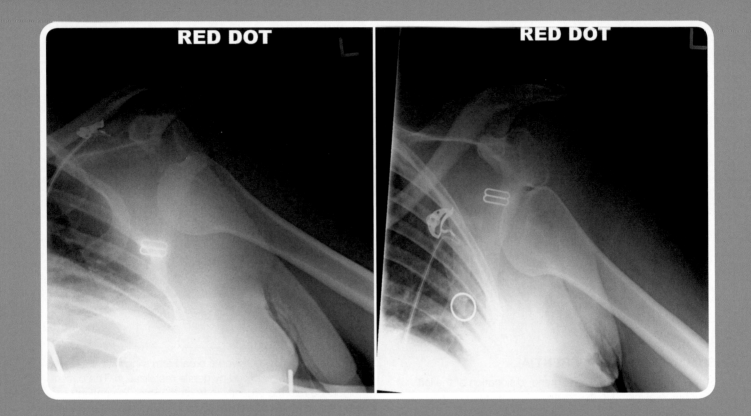

RED DOT RED DOT

TECHNICAL INFORMATION

Patient ID: Anonymous.
Area: Left shoulder.
Projection: AP and apical oblique.
Technical adequacy:

- Adequate coverage.
- Adequate exposure.
- The patient is not rotated.

● FRACTURE DETAILS

There is no fracture.

● JOINTS

There is an anterior dislocation of the left humeral head.

There are no loose bodies.

There is no effusion or lipohaemarthrosis.

There are no arthritic changes.

● SOFT TISSUES

There is no soft tissue swelling.

There is no surgical emphysema.

The imaged left lung is clear.

● BACKGROUND BONE

The background bone is normal.

● BONE LESIONS

There is no bone lesion present.

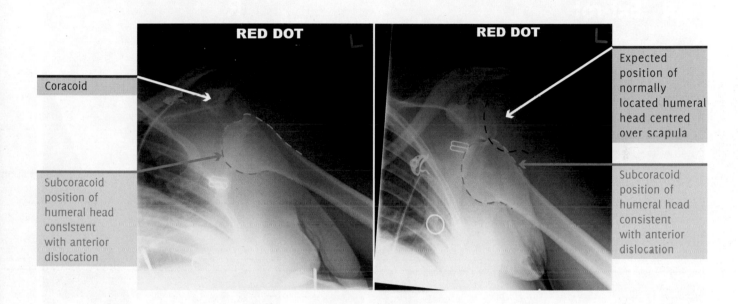

Coracoid

Subcoracoid position of humeral head consistent with anterior dislocation

Expected position of normally located humeral head centred over scapula

Subcoracoid position of humeral head consistent with anterior dislocation

SUMMARY AND DIFFERENTIAL

Both X-rays demonstrate an anterior dislocation of the left glenohumeral joint. No associated humeral head or glenoid fracture is visible.

INVESTIGATIONS AND MANAGEMENT

Advice regarding analgesia should be provided.

The shoulder should undergo closed reduction in the ED under sedation. A check X-ray and repeat neurovascular assessment should be performed.

The arm should be immobilized in a broad arm sling for 2 weeks. After this, the patient should begin gentle mobilization. The patient should be referred to fracture clinic urgently. Over the age of 45 years, there is a high incidence of rotator cuff tear with first-time shoulder dislocations. The patient requires an MRI or ultrasound and consideration for surgery depending on the results.

A 43-year-old man attends his GP because of intermittent pain in his right shoulder, which has persisted for the past several months. He reports that the pain is particularly severe when he is reaching for things in cupboards or high shelves. There is no significant past medical history. On examination, there is a decreased arc of motion, with pain on abduction of the shoulder at 70 to 110 degrees.

X-rays of the right shoulder are requested to assess for a joint abnormality.

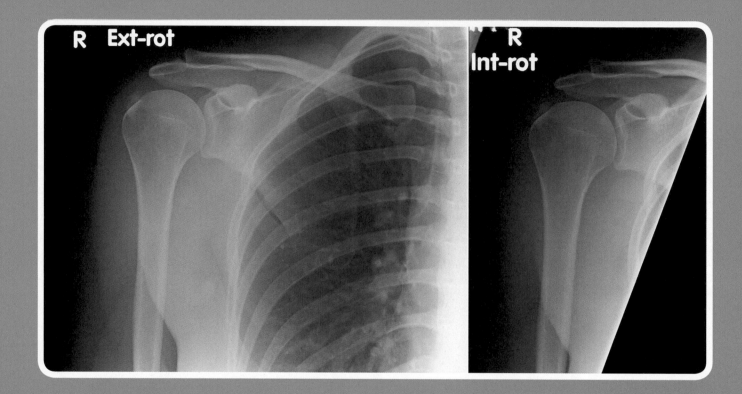

TECHNICAL INFORMATION

Patient ID: Anonymous.
Area: Right shoulder.
Projection: AP external and internal rotation.
Technical adequacy:

- Adequate coverage.
- Adequate exposure.
- Shoulder in internal and external rotation.

● FRACTURE DETAILS

There is no fracture.

● JOINTS

There is no subluxation or dislocation.

There are no loose bodies.

There is no effusion or lipohaemarthrosis.

There are no arthritic changes.

● SOFT TISSUES

There is soft tissue calcification projected over the rotator cuff, at the insertion site of the supraspinatus tendon.

There is no soft tissue swelling.

There is no surgical emphysema.

The visible right lung contains several small calcified nodules. These are likely to be calcified granulomata. The lung is otherwise clear.

● BACKGROUND BONE

The background bone is normal.

● BONE LESIONS

There is no bone lesion present.

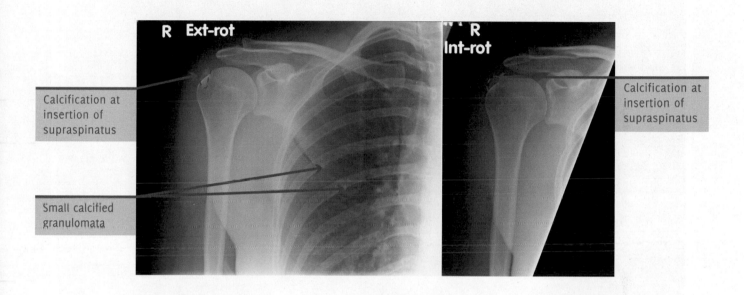

Calcification at insertion of supraspinatus

Small calcified granulomata

Calcification at insertion of supraspinatus

SUMMARY AND DIFFERENTIAL

Findings on these X-rays demonstrate calcification of the supraspinatus tendon. This is in keeping with calcific tendonitis. There is an incidental finding of calcified nodules in the right lung.

INVESTIGATIONS AND MANAGEMENT

Advice regarding analgesia should be provided.

Treatment with NSAIDs and physiotherapy may be provided.

Corticosteroids, needle aspiration and extracorporeal shock-wave therapy can be used (with variable efficacy).

In patients with refractory or progressive symptoms, a referral should be made to an orthopaedic surgeon who may consider operative treatment including arthroscopic subacromial decompression. The calcified granulomata may be related to infection, for example, TB/fungal, and further history/examination should be explored along with a formal chest X-ray.

A 38-year-old male car driver has been brought to a major trauma centre after being involved in an RTC at a combined speed of 45 mph. He was wearing a seatbelt but has been complaining of right shoulder-tip pain since the event. Despite the high energy mechanism of injury, he is triaged to the Minor Injuries Unit and does not have a full ATLS assessment. There is no significant past medical history. On examination, there is full and pain-free range of movement of the right shoulder. Distal pulses are present and motor and sensory function are preserved. The injury is closed.

AP X-rays of the right shoulder are requested to assess for a fracture.

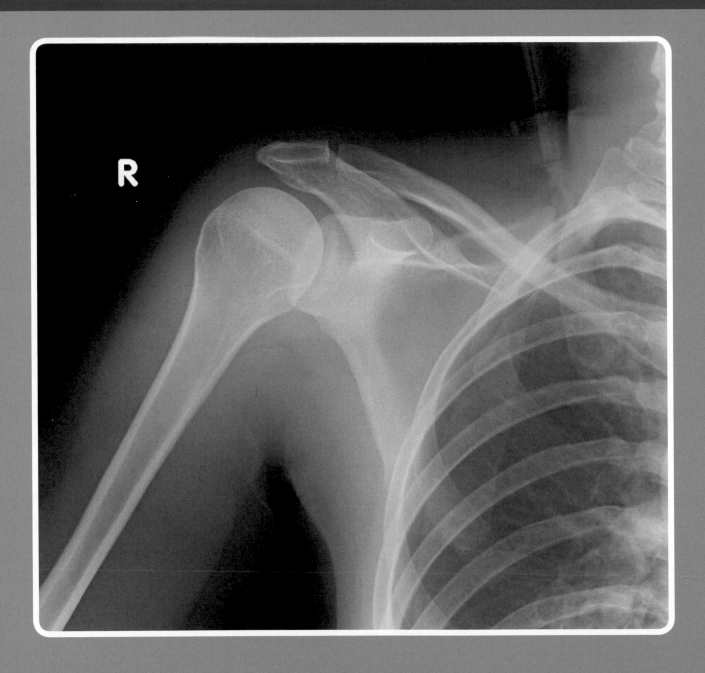

TECHNICAL INFORMATION

Patient ID: Anonymous.
Area: Right shoulder.
Projection: AP.
Technical adequacy:

- Adequate coverage.
- Adequate exposure.
- The patient is not rotated.

● FRACTURE DETAILS

There is no fracture.

● JOINTS

There is no subluxation or dislocation.

There are no loose bodies.

There is no effusion or lipohaemarthrosis.

There are no arthritic changes.

● SOFT TISSUES

There is no soft tissue swelling.

There is no surgical emphysema.

A defined edge can be seen within lung fields of the imaged right lung. Distal to this edge, lung markings are not visible. This is highly likely to be a pneumothorax.

● BACKGROUND BONE

The background bone is normal.

● BONE LESIONS

There is no bone lesion present.

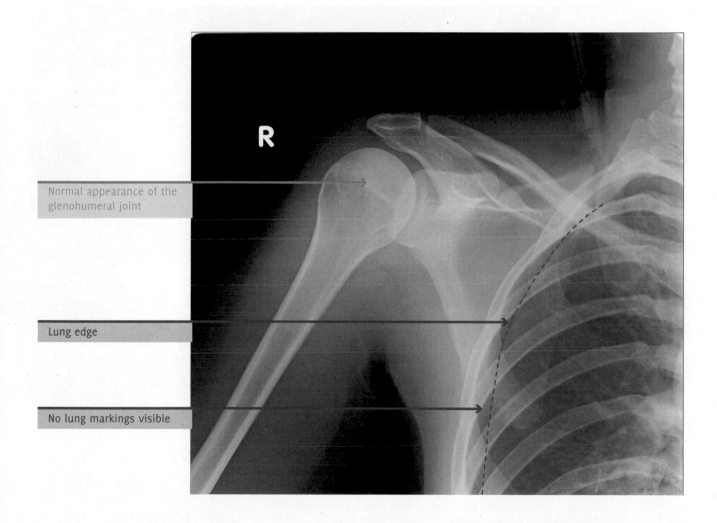

Normal appearance of the glenohumeral joint

Lung edge

No lung markings visible

SUMMARY AND DIFFERENTIAL

This X-ray demonstrates a right-sided pneumothorax. No associated rib fracture is visible.

There is no evidence of proximal humeral fracture or glenohumeral joint dislocation on this single view of the shoulder.

INVESTIGATIONS AND MANAGEMENT

Advice regarding analgesia should be provided.

The patient should be assessed and managed as per ATLS guidelines with triple immobilization, primary and secondary surveys and further imaging depending on the findings to assess for further injury. In most cases, this will be a trauma CT, which is a CT of the head, neck, thorax, abdomen and pelvis with contrast.

Management of the pneumothorax will depend on the size, which is difficult to judge on an incomplete chest X-ray. If it is a small pneumothorax, conservative management would be preferred. A more significant pneumothorax may require aspiration or chest drain insertion.

A 44-year-old builder is brought into the local trauma unit as a trauma call. He has fallen one storey off scaffolding and landed on his left side. He is complaining of pain over the left shoulder. There is no significant past medical history. On examination, there is an abnormal left contour of the shoulder when compared to the right. The patient is tender over the shoulder region. Shoulder movements are minimal and painful. The arm is neurovascularly intact distal to the shoulder. The injury is closed.

AP and Zanca view X-rays of the left shoulder are requested to assess for a fracture.

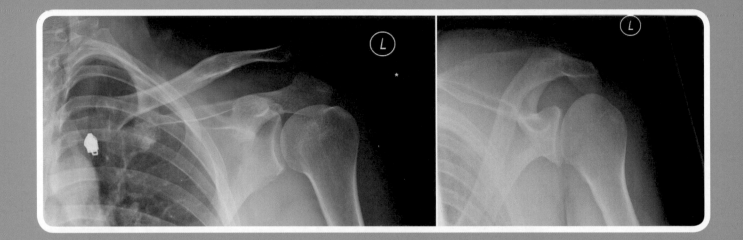

TECHNICAL INFORMATION

Patient ID: Anonymous.
Area: Left shoulder.
Projection: AP and Zanca view.
Technical adequacy:

- Adequate coverage.
- Adequate exposure.
- The patient is not rotated.

● FRACTURE DETAILS

There is no fracture.

● JOINTS

There is acromioclavicular joint disruption, with elevation of the distal clavicle above the level of the acromion and marked widening of the coracoclavicular distance (>25 mm).

There is no subluxation or dislocation of the glenohumeral joint.

There are no loose bodies.

There is no effusion or lipohaemarthrosis.

There are no arthritic changes.

● SOFT TISSUES

There is no skin tenting present.

There is no soft tissue swelling.

There is no surgical emphysema.

The imaged left lung apex is clear.

● BACKGROUND BONE

The background bone is normal.

● BONE LESIONS

There is no bone lesion present.

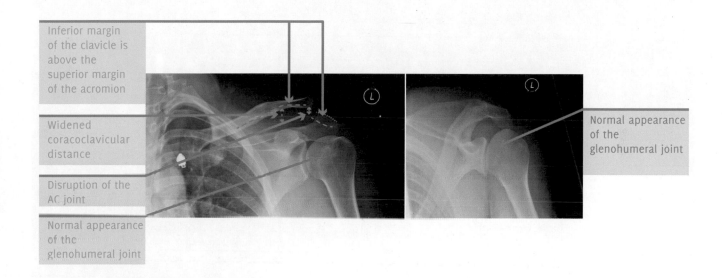

Inferior margin of the clavicle is above the superior margin of the acromion

Widened coracoclavicular distance

Disruption of the AC joint

Normal appearance of the glenohumeral joint

Normal appearance of the glenohumeral joint

SUMMARY AND DIFFERENTIAL

Both X-rays demonstrate disruption of the left acromioclavicular joint. The elevated clavicle above the level of the acromion and the markedly widened coracoclavicular distance are consistent with a Rockwood grade 5 acromioclavicular joint injury. There is no glenohumeral dislocation or fracture.

INVESTIGATIONS AND MANAGEMENT

Advice regarding analgesia should be provided.

The patient should be assessed as per ATLS guidelines.

A collar and cuff should be fitted for comfort.

A referral should be made to an orthopaedic surgeon who may consider ORIF and/or ligament reconstruction.

An 18-year-old man fell from his mountain bike onto his left shoulder. He has been driven to the nearest ED by a friend. There is no significant past medical history. On examination, there is a reduced range of movement at the left shoulder, with pain at the lateral portion of the clavicle and an obvious deformity at the ACJ. Distal pulses are present and sensory and motor function is preserved, including specifically the axillary nerve. The injury is closed.

An AP X-ray of the left ACJ is requested to assess for fracture.

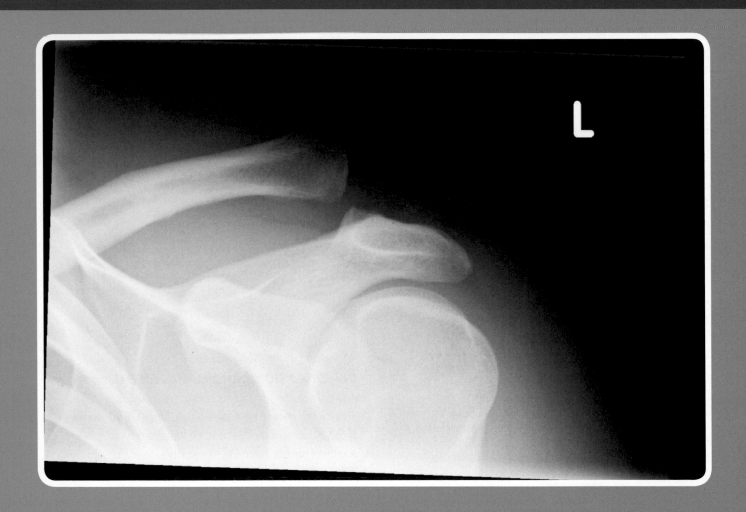

TECHNICAL INFORMATION

Patient ID: Anonymous.
Area: Left acromioclavicular joint.
Projection: AP.
Technical adequacy:

- Adequate coverage.
- Adequate exposure.
- The patient is not rotated.

● FRACTURE DETAILS

There is no fracture.

● JOINTS

There is ACJ disruption, with elevation of the distal clavicle above the level of the acromion and marked widening of the coracoclavicular distance (>25 mm).

There are no loose bodies.

There is no effusion or lipohaemarthrosis.

There are no arthritic changes.

● SOFT TISSUES

There is deformity of the distal clavicle displacing the soft tissues.

There is no surgical emphysema.

The imaged lung apex is clear.

● BACKGROUND BONE

The background bone is normal.

● BONE LESIONS

There is no bone lesion present.

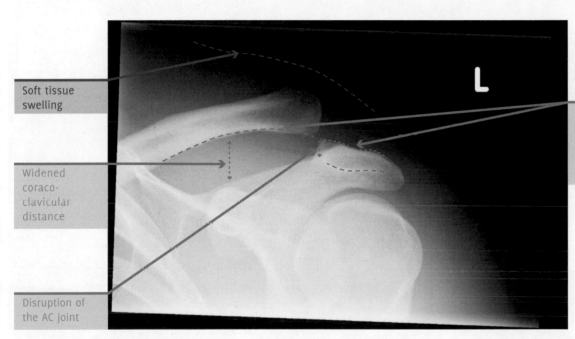

Soft tissue swelling

Widened coraco-clavicular distance

Disruption of the AC joint

Inferior margin of the clavicle is above the superior margin of the acromion

SUMMARY AND DIFFERENTIAL

This X-ray demonstrates dislocation of the ACJ. The combination of marked clavicular elevation (above the level of the acromion) and markedly widened coracoclavicular distance is consistent with a significant ACJ injury.

INVESTIGATIONS AND MANAGEMENT

Appropriate analgesia should be provided.

A broad arm sling should be fitted for comfort.

A referral should be made to an orthopaedic surgeon who may consider ORIF and potential repair of ligaments.

A 26-year-old man has fallen from his scooter onto his right shoulder. He has been brought into the ED as a trauma call. There is no significant past medical history. On examination, there is a deformity over the middle of the clavicle. Distal pulses are present and sensory and motor function is preserved, including specifically the axillary nerve. The injury is closed.

An AP X-ray of the right clavicle is requested to assess for fracture.

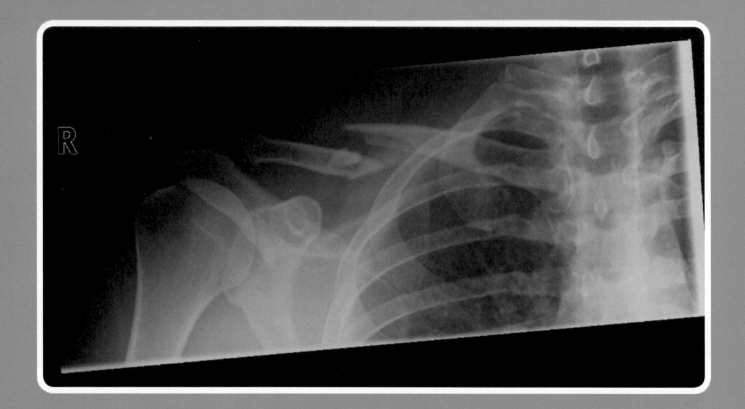

TECHNICAL INFORMATION

Patient ID: Anonymous.
Area: Right clavicle.
Projection: AP.
Technical adequacy:

- Adequate coverage.
- Adequate exposure but series should include 15- and 45-degree views to assess for displacement.
- The patient is not rotated.

● FRACTURE DETAILS

There is a fracture of the middle third of the clavicle.

The fracture is transverse, comminuted and extraarticular.

The distal clavicle is inferiorly displaced in relation to the proximal clavicle.

There is inferior angulation at the fracture site.

There is no rotation evident on this single view.

There is some shortening present.

● JOINTS

There is no subluxation or dislocation. In particular, the ACJ alignment and coracoclavicular distance are normal.

There are no loose bodies.

There is no effusion or lipohaemarthrosis.

There are no arthritic changes.

● SOFT TISSUES

There is no soft tissue swelling.

There is no surgical emphysema.

The imaged lung apex is clear.

● BACKGROUND BONE

The background bone is normal.

● BONE LESIONS

There is no bone lesion present.

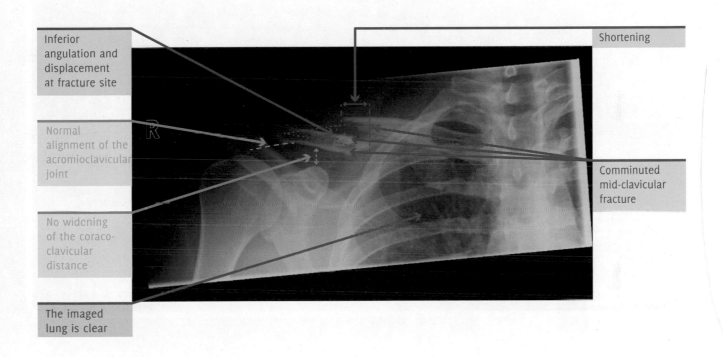

Inferior angulation and displacement at fracture site

Normal alignment of the acromioclavicular joint

No widening of the coraco-clavicular distance

The imaged lung is clear

Shortening

Comminuted mid-clavicular fracture

SUMMARY AND DIFFERENTIAL

This X-ray demonstrates a comminuted mid-clavicular fracture with angulation, marked displacement and shortening.

INVESTIGATIONS AND MANAGEMENT

Appropriate analgesia should be provided.

A broad arm sling should be fitted for comfort.

A referral to an orthopaedic surgeon to consider ORIF should be made, as this is a high-energy injury with comminution, shortening and displacement, increasing the risk of nonunion or reduced long-term shoulder function with nonoperative treatment.

A 25-year-old woman has fallen from a trampoline onto her left shoulder and attends a Minor Injuries Unit. There is no significant past medical history. On examination, the patient is tender over the left ACJ. There is a good range of movement of the glenohumeral joint. Distal pulses are present and sensory and motor function including specifically the axillary nerve is preserved. The injury is closed.

An AP X-ray of the left clavicle is requested to assess for fracture.

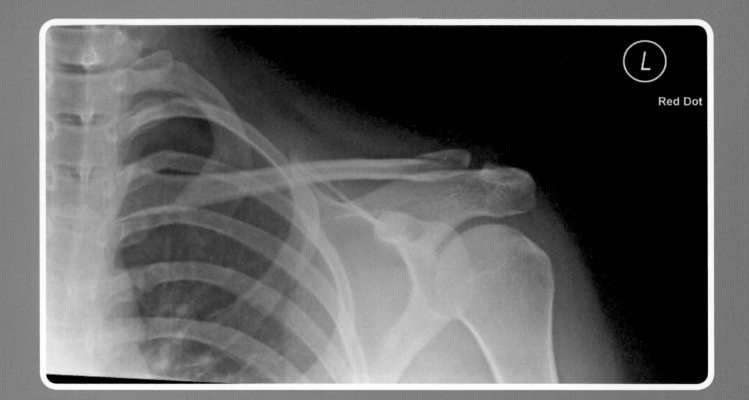

L

Red Dot

TECHNICAL INFORMATION

Patient ID: Anonymous.
Area: Left clavicle.
Projection: AP.
Technical adequacy:

- Adequate coverage.
- Adequate exposure.
- The patient is not rotated.

● FRACTURE DETAILS

There is a fracture of the distal third of the clavicle.

The fracture is oblique, simple and intraarticular.

There is minimal displacement on this view.

There is no angulation.

There is no rotation.

There is no shortening.

● JOINTS

There is no subluxation or dislocation. In particular, the ACJ alignment and coracoclavicular distance are normal.

There are no loose bodies.

There is no effusion or lipohaemarthrosis.

There are no arthritic changes.

● SOFT TISSUES

There is no soft tissue swelling.

There is no surgical emphysema.

The imaged lung apex is clear.

● BACKGROUND BONE

The background bone is normal.

● BONE LESIONS

There is no bone lesion present.

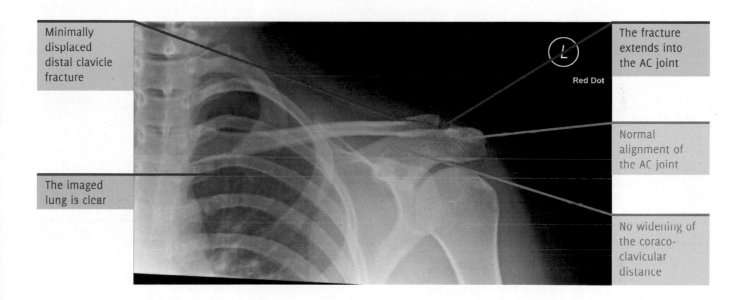

Minimally displaced distal clavicle fracture

The imaged lung is clear

Red Dot

The fracture extends into the AC joint

Normal alignment of the AC joint

No widening of the coraco-clavicular distance

SUMMARY AND DIFFERENTIAL

This X-ray demonstrates a minimally displaced fracture involving the distal third of the clavicle with extension into the ACJ. The minimal displacement suggests the coracoclavicular ligaments are intact. This suggests that the fracture is stable, with a high likelihood of achieving union with nonoperative means.

INVESTIGATIONS AND MANAGEMENT

Appropriate analgesia should be provided.

Further imaging should be completed (the series should include 15- and 45-degree views to assess for displacement).

A broad arm sling should be fitted.

The patient should be referred to fracture clinic. The fracture will most likely be treated nonoperatively with early gentle ROM exercises and follow-up at around 6 weeks to confirm union.

A referral should be made to physiotherapy.

An 83-year-old woman has been brought into the ED by her daughter. She lost her balance whilst hoovering at home and fell directly backwards onto her back. She has been complaining of mid-back pain since and has been struggling to walk. She has a past medical history of osteoporosis. On examination, there is kyphosis of the spine. The patient is tender para-spinally and over the spinal processes of the thoraco-lumbar junction. On examination of the lower limbs, no abnormal neurology is elicited. PR exam reveals normal tone and squeeze. A postvoid bladder scan reveals no residual urine volume. The injury is closed.

AP and lateral X-rays of the thoracic spine are requested to assess for a fracture.

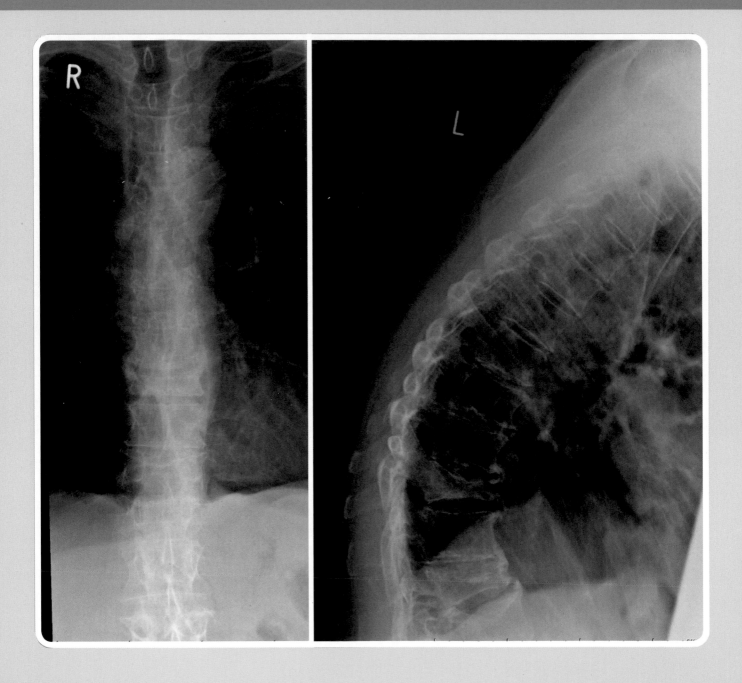

TECHNICAL INFORMATION

Patient ID: Anonymous.
Area: Thoracic spine.
Projection: AP and lateral.
Technical adequacy:

- Adequate coverage.
- Adequate exposure.
- The patient is not rotated.

● FRACTURE DETAILS

There are compression fractures involving the T10 and T12 vertebrae.

The fractures do not appear to involve the posterior elements of the vertebrae.

A minimum of 50% loss of height of the anterior margin of the vertebral body is observed.

There is a superior endplate fracture of L1.

The fracture does not appear to involve the posterior elements.

● JOINTS

There is increased thoracic kyphosis related to the lower thoracic wedge compression fractures. Vertebral alignment is otherwise normal.

There is no subluxation or dislocation.

There are no loose bodies.

There is no effusion or lipohaemarthrosis.

Arthritic changes are visible, with anterolateral osteophyte formation in the lower thoracic and upper lumbar spine.

● SOFT TISSUES

There is no soft tissue swelling.

There is no surgical emphysema.

The partially imaged lung is clear.

● BACKGROUND BONE

The background bone is diffusely osteopenic.

● BONE LESIONS

There is no bone lesion present.

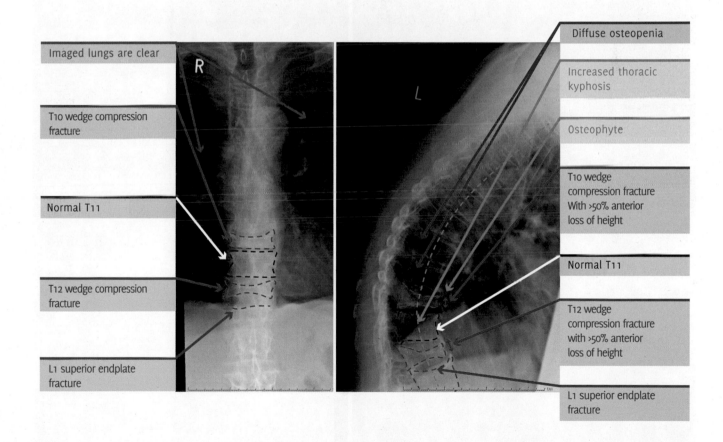

Imaged lungs are clear

T10 wedge compression fracture

Normal T11

T12 wedge compression fracture

L1 superior endplate fracture

Diffuse osteopenia

Increased thoracic kyphosis

Osteophyte

T10 wedge compression fracture With >50% anterior loss of height

Normal T11

T12 wedge compression fracture with >50% anterior loss of height

L1 superior endplate fracture

SUMMARY AND DIFFERENTIAL

Both X-rays demonstrate osteoporotic type vertebral fractures. Specifically, there are T10 and T12 wedge fractures with marked loss of anterior height. The fractures do not appear to involve the posterior elements and are therefore considered stable. There is also a superior endplate fracture of L1.

INVESTIGATIONS AND MANAGEMENT

Advice regarding analgesia should be provided.

A CT scan should be performed to further assess the extent of the injury and a referral made to a tertiary spinal service for an opinion. It is likely these are stable fractures, which can be treated nonoperatively.

If symptomatic, a TLSO brace should be fitted and the patient be referred to physiotherapy to maximize mobility.

Osteoporosis should be investigated and treated if this has not been done already.

A 27-year-old woman is referred to the ED by her GP as she has been suffering with lower back pain for several weeks following a fall down two stairs at home. The pain is exacerbated by long periods of standing and she is struggling to mobilize when walking up stairs. There is no significant past medical history. On examination, there is pain on deep palpation at the base of the lumbar spine.

AP and lateral X-rays of the lumbosacral spine are requested to exclude a fracture.

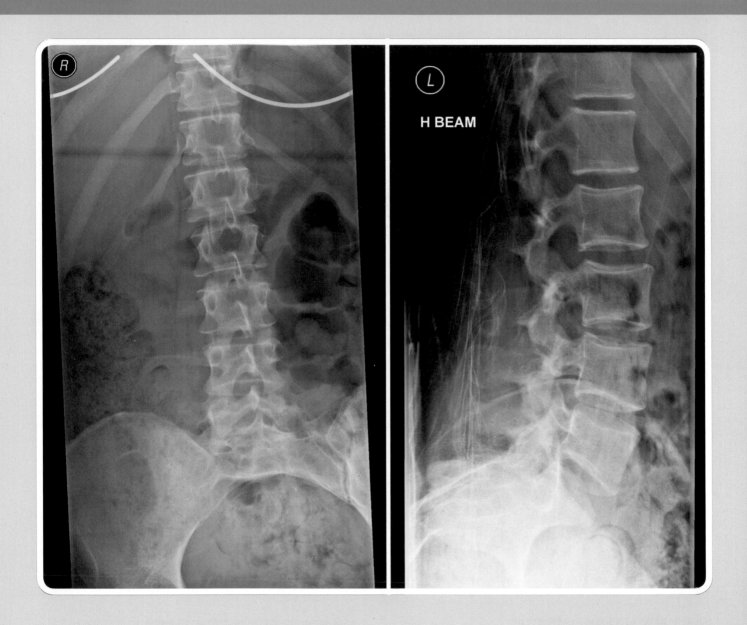

TECHNICAL INFORMATION

Patient ID: Anonymous.
Area: Lumbosacral spine.
Projection: AP and lateral.
Technical adequacy:

- Adequate coverage.
- Adequate exposure.
- The patient is not rotated.

● FRACTURE DETAILS

There is no fracture.

● JOINTS

There is sclerosis of the right SI joint with complete obliteration of the joint space. The left SI joint is normal.

Vertebral alignment is normal.

There is no subluxation or dislocation.

● SOFT TISSUES

There is no soft tissue swelling.

There is no surgical emphysema.

Psoas outlines are preserved.

The imaged bowel gas pattern is normal.

● BACKGROUND BONE

The background bone is normal.

● BONE LESIONS

There is no bone lesion present.

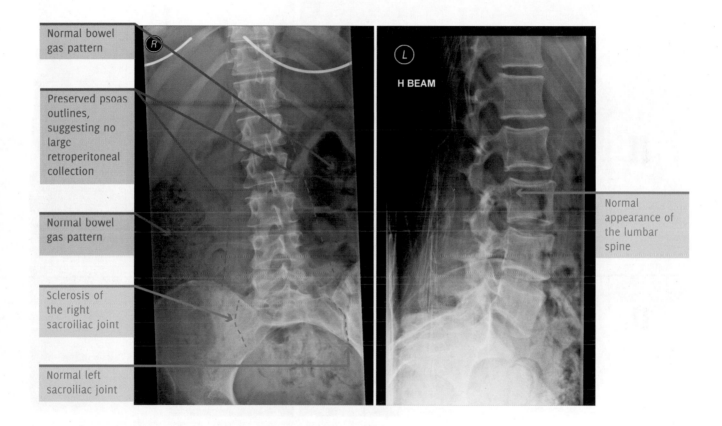

Normal bowel gas pattern

Preserved psoas outlines, suggesting no large retroperitoneal collection

Normal bowel gas pattern

Sclerosis of the right sacroiliac joint

Normal left sacroiliac joint

H BEAM

Normal appearance of the lumbar spine

SUMMARY AND DIFFERENTIAL

Both X-rays demonstrate right SI joint sacroiliitis. The differential diagnosis for unilateral sacroiliitis includes ankylosing spondylitis and septic arthritis. Given the patient has no destructive features on X-ray and is systemically well, a spondyloarthropathy is more likely.

INVESTIGATIONS AND MANAGEMENT

Advice regarding analgesia should be provided.

Blood tests for inflammatory markers should be sent. An MRI scan should be requested to further delineate the SI joint and, in particular, assess for evidence of osteomyelitis or any associated soft tissue abscess, for example, involvement of the iliac or psoas muscles.

A 33-year-old window cleaner has been brought into the local trauma unit as a trauma call. He has fallen off his ladder at a height of approximately 10 feet. He describes striking the back of his head on the ground. After a full primary and secondary survey, he is found to be complaining of neck pain, but has had no loss of consciousness. There is no significant past medical history. On examination, the patient is tender over the cervical spine, with pain on all movements. There is no neurological deficit in the upper or lower limbs. The injury is closed.

AP and lateral X-rays of the cervical spine and a peg view are requested to assess for a fracture.

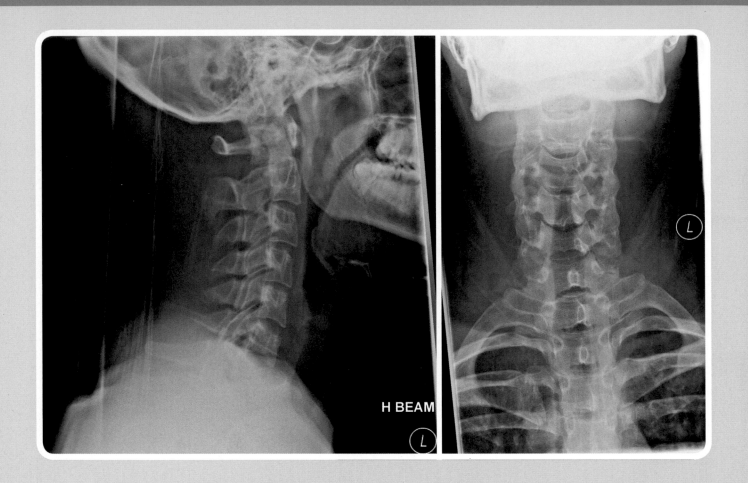

TECHNICAL INFORMATION

Patient ID: Anonymous.
Area: Cervical spine.
Projection: AP, lateral and peg views.
Technical adequacy:

- Inadequate coverage – the C6/7 and C7/T1 disc spaces are not visible on the lateral view.
- Adequate exposure.
- The patient is rotated on the lateral view.

● FRACTURE DETAILS

There is no fracture.

● JOINTS

The alignment of the spinous processes on the AP view is abnormal at C6/7. There is also widening of the interspinous space at C6/7 on the lateral view. These findings are consistent with a unilateral C6/7 facet joint dislocation.

Vertebral alignment is otherwise normal in the imaged cervical spine.

There are no arthritic changes.

● SOFT TISSUES

There is no swelling of the prevertebral soft tissues.

There is no surgical emphysema.

The imaged lung apices are clear.

Artefact from the hard collar is visible.

● BACKGROUND BONE

The background bone is normal.

● BONE LESIONS

There is no bone lesion present.

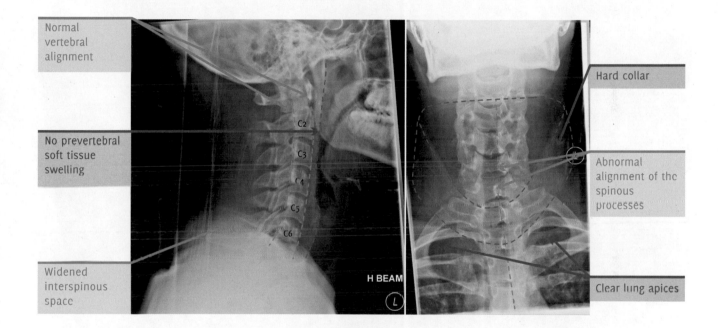

SUMMARY AND DIFFERENTIAL

Both X-rays demonstrate a C6/7 unilateral facet joint dislocation.

INVESTIGATIONS AND MANAGEMENT

Advice regarding analgesia should be provided.

The patient should be managed as per ATLS protocol.

A noncontrast CT of the cervical spine should be obtained for further assessment of the injury.

A referral should be made to a spinal surgeon for further management, which may include MRI, closed or open reduction and surgical stabilization.

A 35-year-old male presents to the spine/back clinic because of a gradual onset of lower back pain and stiffness over the past 10 months. He reports that the pain and stiffness are worse in the morning. His symptoms are also worsened by standing for long periods of time and when walking up stairs. There is no significant past medical history. On examination, there is decreased lumbar spine flexion, positive Schober's test and a Faber's test is positive bilaterally.

AP and lateral X-rays of the lumbosacral spine are requested to assess for alignment and a fracture.

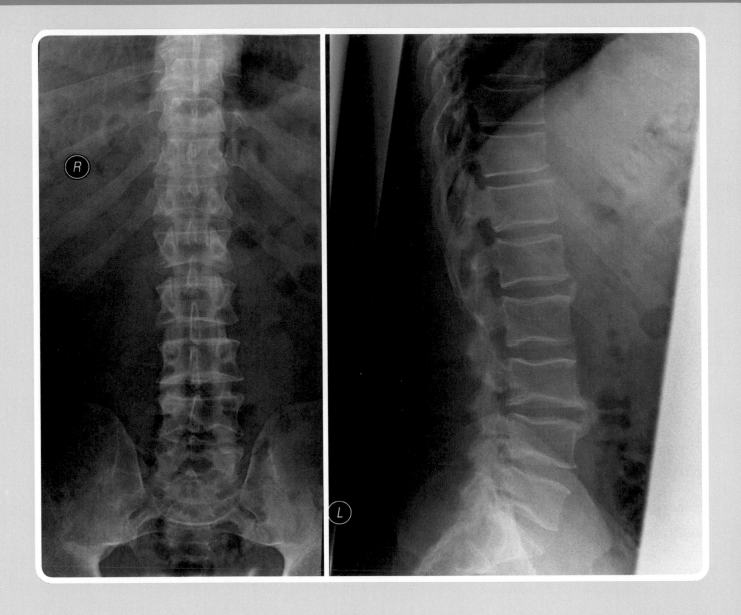

TECHNICAL INFORMATION

Patient ID: Anonymous.
Area: Lumbosacral spine.
Projection: AP and lateral.
Technical adequacy:

- Adequate coverage.
- Adequate exposure.
- The patient is not rotated.

● FRACTURE DETAILS

There is no fracture.

● JOINTS

There are degenerative changes with sclerosis and loss of joint space of the bilateral SI joints.

Vertebral alignment is normal.

There is no subluxation or dislocation.

Arthritic changes can be seen in the spine, with anterior nonmarginal osteophyte formation at L1/2 and L3/4.

● SOFT TISSUES

There is no soft tissue swelling.

There is no surgical emphysema.

Psoas outlines are preserved.

The imaged bowel gas pattern is normal.

● BACKGROUND BONE

The background bone is normal.

● BONE LESIONS

There is no bone lesion present.

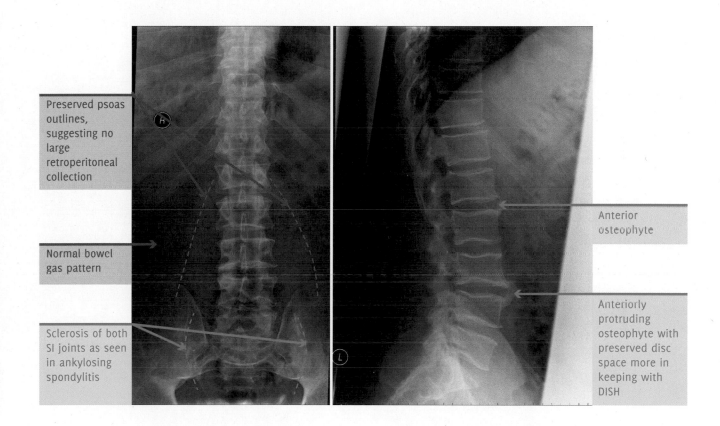

Preserved psoas outlines, suggesting no large retroperitoneal collection

Normal bowel gas pattern

Sclerosis of both SI joints as seen in ankylosing spondylitis

Anterior osteophyte

Anteriorly protruding osteophyte with preserved disc space more in keeping with DISH

SUMMARY AND DIFFERENTIAL

Both X-rays demonstrate bilateral symmetrical sacroiliitis. Ankylosing spondylitis is the most likely aetiology, given the clinical history of progressive stiffness and pain. Importantly, sacroiliitis is usually the first manifestation of ankylosing spondylitis. The differential diagnosis for these X-ray appearances also includes enteropathic arthritis and DISH. The lumbar spine appearances are more characteristic of DISH as the disc spaces are preserved and osteophytes protrude anteriorly.

INVESTIGATIONS AND MANAGEMENT

Advice regarding analgesia should be provided.

The patient can be managed nonoperatively with NSAIDs and physiotherapy.

The underlying systemic disease should be investigated and treated.

HIP AND PELVIS

An 87-year-old female nursing home resident fell over while attempting to reach the toilet at night. She has been brought to the ED by ambulance. She has a past medical history of hypertension, diabetes and mild cognitive impairment. On examination, the right leg is shortened and externally rotated. Distal pulses are present and sensory and motor function is preserved. The injury is closed.

AP and lateral X-rays of the right hip are requested to assess for fracture.

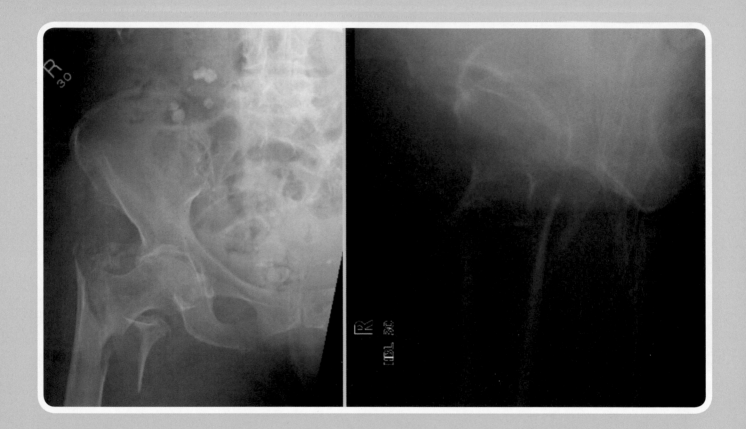

TECHNICAL INFORMATION

Patient ID: Anonymous.
Area: Right hip.
Projection: AP and lateral.
Technical adequacy:

- Adequate coverage.
- Adequate exposure.
- The patient is not rotated.

● FRACTURE DETAILS

There is a fracture involving the intertrochanteric neck of femur.

The fracture is oblique, three-part comminuted and extraarticular.

There is posterior displacement of the main fracture fragment.

There is varus angulation. The neck shaft angle is approximately 110 degrees (normal is 125–130 degrees).

There is external rotation.

There is shortening.

● JOINTS

There is no subluxation or dislocation.

There are no loose bodies.

There is no effusion or lipohaemarthrosis.

There are arthritic changes at the right hip joint with loss of joint space and subchondral sclerosis.

● SOFT TISSUES

There is no soft tissue swelling.

There is no surgical emphysema.

● BACKGROUND BONE

The background bone is osteopenic.

● BONE LESIONS

There is no bone lesion present.

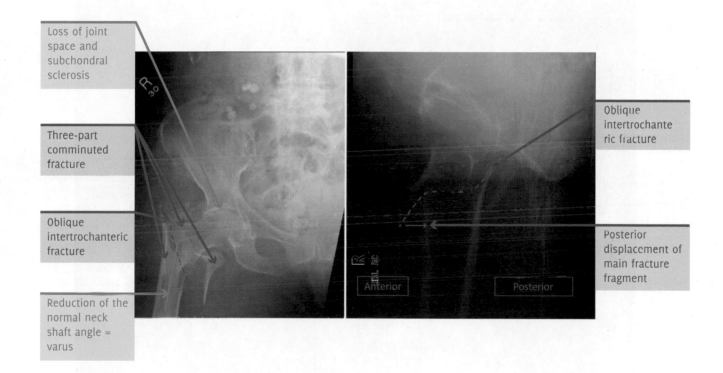

Loss of joint space and subchondral sclerosis

Three-part comminuted fracture

Oblique intertrochanteric fracture

Reduction of the normal neck shaft angle = varus

Oblique intertrochanteric fracture

Posterior displacement of main fracture fragment

Anterior

Posterior

SUMMARY AND DIFFERENTIAL

These X-rays demonstrate a three-part comminuted right-sided extracapsular neck of femur fracture on a background of arthritic changes and osteopenic bone.

INVESTIGATIONS AND MANAGEMENT

Appropriate analgesia should be provided.

The patient should be managed by a multidisciplinary team including orthogeriatricians who specialize in the management of hip fracture patients. As part of this treatment, a referral should be made to an orthopaedic surgeon for operative fixation with a dynamic hip screw or an intramedullary nail, as nearly all hip fractures require surgical management.

An 82-year-old woman slipped in the bathroom while getting out of the shower, landing on her right side. She usually mobilizes independently. She has a past medical history of osteoporosis (on bisphosphonates), hypertension, angina, myocardial infarction and TIA. On examination, the patient has a painful right proximal femur and is unable to mobilize. Distal pulses are present and sensory and motor function is preserved. The injury is closed.

AP and lateral X-rays of the right hip are requested to assess for a fracture.

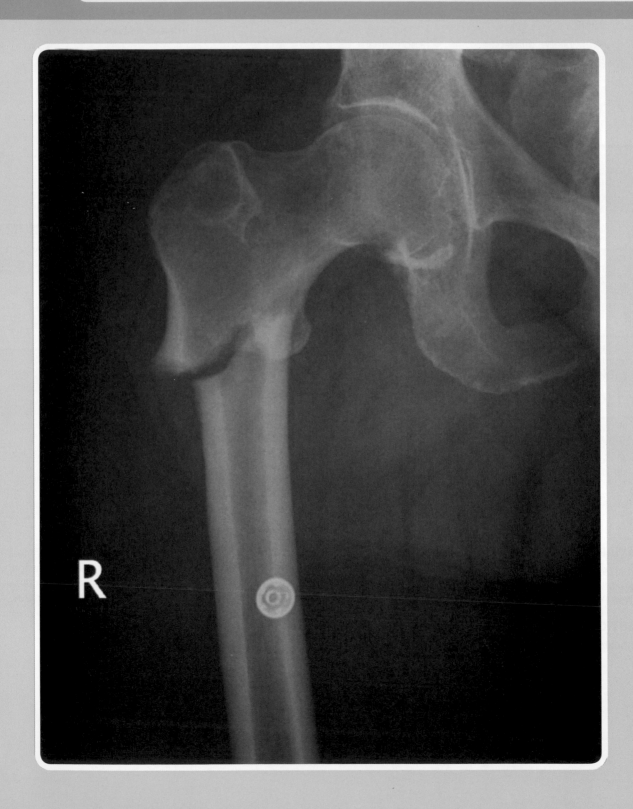

TECHNICAL INFORMATION

Patient ID: Anonymous.
Area: Right hip.
Projection: AP.
Technical adequacy:

- Inadequate coverage – the AP view does not fully include the pubic rami, and no lateral view is present.
- Adequate exposure.
- The patient is not rotated.

● FRACTURE DETAILS

There is a fracture involving the proximal femur, adjacent and distal to the lesser trochanter.

The fracture is oblique, simple and extraarticular.

There is displacement with mild varus angulation.

There is no rotation.

There is no shortening.

● JOINTS

There is no subluxation or dislocation.

There are no loose bodies.

There is no effusion or lipohaemarthrosis.

There are arthritic changes present in the right hip, with joint space narrowing and subchondral sclerosis.

● SOFT TISSUES

There is no soft tissue swelling.

There is no surgical emphysema.

● BACKGROUND BONE

The lateral cortex at the fracture site appears hypertrophic.

● BONE LESIONS

There is no bone lesion present.

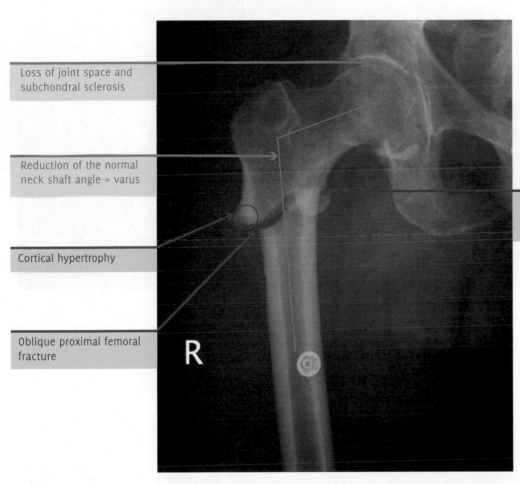

Loss of joint space and subchondral sclerosis

Reduction of the normal neck shaft angle = varus

Cortical hypertrophy

Oblique proximal femoral fracture

The fracture is adjacent and distal to the lesser trochanter

R

SUMMARY AND DIFFERENTIAL

These X-rays demonstrate a subtrochanteric femoral fracture. The cortical thickening around the fracture site suggests this is a pathological fracture secondary to bisphosphonate therapy.

INVESTIGATIONS AND MANAGEMENT

Appropriate analgesia should be provided.

A full AP X-ray should be requested, including the whole pubic rami.

The patient should be managed by a multidisciplinary team including orthogeriatricians who specialize in the management of hip fracture patients. As part of this treatment, a referral should be made to an orthopaedic surgeon for operative fixation with an intramedullary nail. Intraoperative bone samples should be sent to the lab for histology to exclude metastatic disease as a cause for the fracture.

A 71-year-old woman presents to the ED after developing sudden onset severe right-hip pain on bending over to pick something up. She reports also hearing a 'pop' sound. The patient has had a previous right total hip replacement and left Girdlestone procedure. On examination, the patient is unable to actively move her hip. The right leg is externally rotated and held in extension. The right leg appears longer than the left. Distal pulses are present and motor and sensory function is preserved.

AP pelvis and lateral right-hip X-rays are requested to assess for fracture.

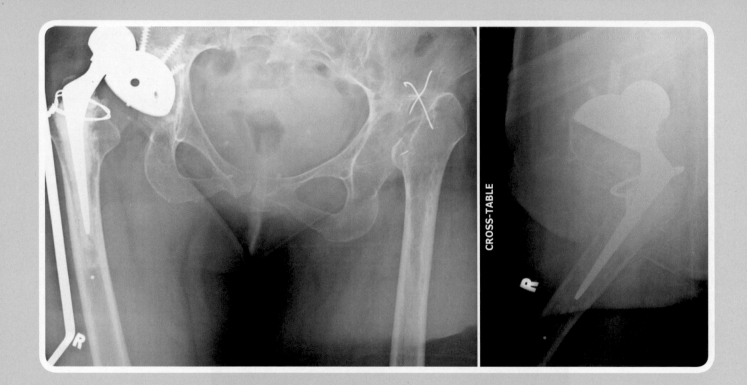

CROSS-TABLE

R

TECHNICAL INFORMATION

Patient ID: Anonymous.
Area: Pelvis and right hip.
Projection: AP and lateral.
Technical adequacy:

- Adequate coverage.
- Adequate exposure.
- The patient is not rotated.

● FRACTURE DETAILS

There is no fracture.

● JOINTS

There is an anterior dislocation of the right total hip replacement. There is a suspicion of a lucent line around the acetabular component, which has been placed superiorly. The femoral component is cemented without any osteolysis, but the greater trochanter is no longer visible and there is a cable superior to the lesser trochanter.

There are no loose bodies.

There is no effusion or lipohaemarthrosis.

There are no arthritic changes.

● SOFT TISSUES

There is no soft tissue swelling.

There is no surgical emphysema.

● BACKGROUND BONE

There is a previous left Girdlestone procedure. The background bone is otherwise normal.

● BONE LESIONS

There is no bone lesion present.

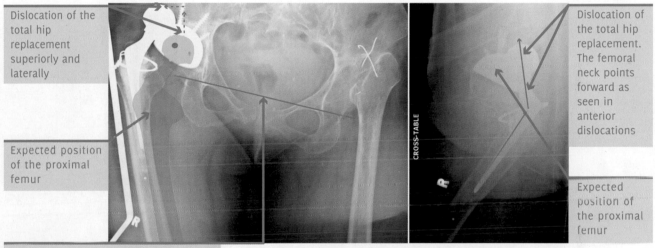

Dislocation of the total hip replacement superiorly and laterally

Expected position of the proximal femur

The lesser trochanter is higher on the left demonstrating that despite the dislocation the left leg is still shorter as a result of the girdlestone (excision of the hip joint)

CROSS-TABLE

Dislocation of the total hip replacement. The femoral neck points forward as seen in anterior dislocations

Expected position of the proximal femur

SUMMARY AND DIFFERENTIAL

These X-rays demonstrate an anterior dislocation of the right total hip replacement.

INVESTIGATIONS AND MANAGEMENT

Appropriate analgesia should be provided.

The hip should be reduced under sedation or general anaesthetic. The patient should be referred to orthopaedics who may investigate the cause of dislocation and consider surgical intervention if this is a recurrent problem in a patient fit for surgery.

A 74-year-old gentleman presents to the ED having tripped over his garden step, landing on his right side. He has a past medical history of a right total hip replacement for osteoarthritis and a left dynamic hip screw. On examination, the patient is unable to mobilize. There is a painful right hip, with bruising over the thigh. Distal pulses are present. Sensory and motor function is preserved. The injury is closed.

AP pelvis and lateral right-hip X-rays are requested to assess for fracture.

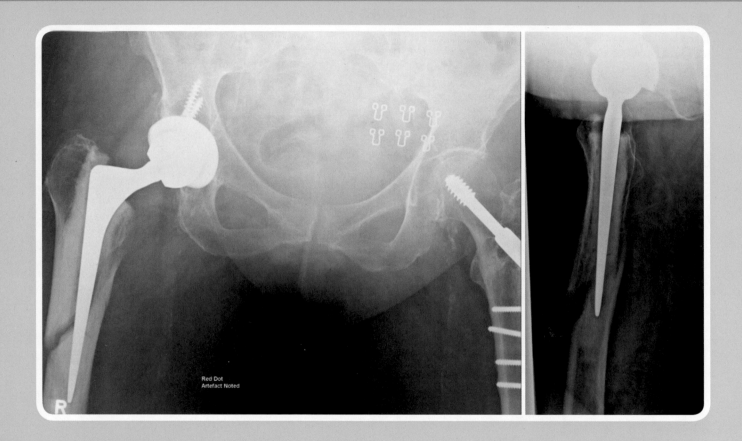

Red Dot
Artefact Noted

TECHNICAL INFORMATION

Patient ID: Anonymous.
Area: Right hip.
Projection: AP pelvis and lateral right hip.
Technical adequacy:

- Adequate coverage.
- Adequate exposure.
- The patient is not rotated.

● FRACTURE DETAILS

There is a fracture involving the femoral shaft. It is adjacent to the femoral component of the right total hip replacement.

The fracture is spiral, simple and extraarticular.

There is minimal posterior and medial displacement.

There is minimal posterior angulation.

There is no rotation.

There is no shortening.

There is some lucency around the femoral component of the right total hip replacement.

● JOINTS

There is no subluxation or dislocation.

There are no loose bodies.

There is no effusion or lipohaemarthrosis.

There are no arthritic changes.

● SOFT TISSUES

There is no soft tissue swelling.

There is no surgical emphysema.

There is vascular calcification.

● BACKGROUND BONE

The background bone appears osteopenic.

● BONE LESIONS

There is no bone lesion present.

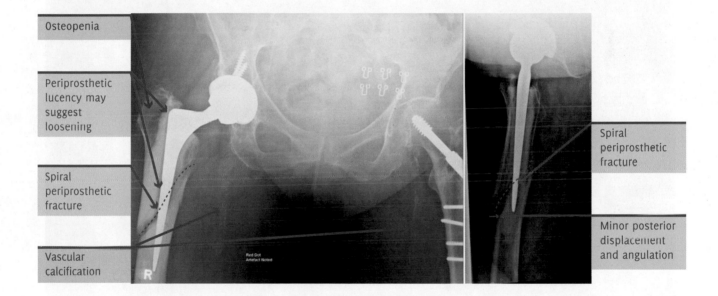

Osteopenia

Periprosthetic lucency may suggest loosening

Spiral periprosthetic fracture

Vascular calcification

Red Dot
Artefact Noted

R

Spiral periprosthetic fracture

Minor posterior displacement and angulation

SUMMARY AND DIFFERENTIAL

These X-rays demonstrate a periprosthetic femoral shaft fracture with fracture of the cement mantle and a loose femoral implant.

INVESTIGATIONS AND MANAGEMENT

Appropriate analgesia should be provided.

A referral should be made to the orthopaedic team. There are several options for management. Surgery may involve removing the loose implant and stabilizing the fracture with a plate. This may be followed by performing a 'cement in cement' revision where a new slightly smaller implant is used along with new cement. The old cement is left in situ.

A 69-year-old woman presents to hip clinic. She complains of severely painful hips and difficulty mobilizing. She reports the right hip is worse but that the problem is bilateral. There is no significant past medical history. On examination, the patient walks with an antalgic gait. There is a reduced range of movement caused by pain. Pain is reproduced by flexion and internal rotation. There is a fixed flexion deformity on the right side. Distal pulses are present and sensory and motor function is preserved.

An AP X-ray of the pelvis is requested to assess for degenerative changes.

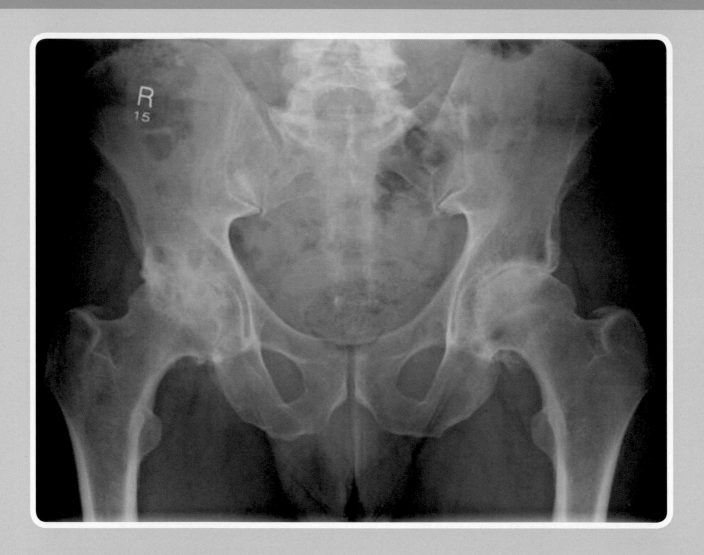

TECHNICAL INFORMATION

Patient ID: Anonymous.
Area: Pelvis.
Projection: AP.
Technical adequacy:

- Adequate coverage.
- Adequate exposure.
- The patient is not rotated.

● FRACTURE DETAILS

There is no fracture.

● JOINTS

There is no subluxation or dislocation.

There are no loose bodies.

There is no effusion or lipohaemarthrosis.

There are arthritic changes affecting both hip joints. On the left, there is almost complete loss of joint space, subchondral sclerosis and osteophyte formation.

On the right, there is complete loss of joint space, subchondral sclerosis and subchondral cysts with osteophyte formation.

● SOFT TISSUES

There is no soft tissue swelling.

There is no surgical emphysema.

● BACKGROUND BONE

The background bone is normal.

● BONE LESIONS

There is no bone lesion present.

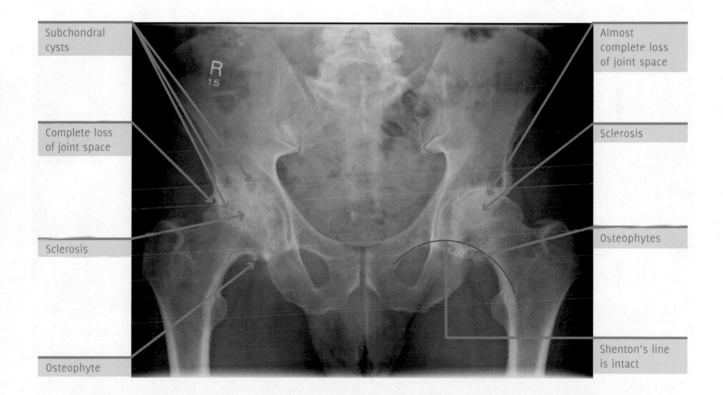

Subchondral cysts

Complete loss of joint space

Sclerosis

Osteophyte

Almost complete loss of joint space

Sclerosis

Osteophytes

Shenton's line is intact

SUMMARY AND DIFFERENTIAL

This X-ray demonstrates severe right-hip degenerative changes alongside moderate to severe left-hip degenerative changes.

INVESTIGATIONS AND MANAGEMENT

Appropriate analgesia should be provided.

The patient should be given advice regarding lifestyle modification to control weight and minimize extra stress on weight-bearing joints, as well as information on walking aids if appropriate.

A referral should be made to an orthopaedic surgeon who may consider a THR.

An 82-year-old male fell over whilst carrying out the bins. He has since been unable to mobilize and has been brought to the ED by ambulance. He usually mobilizes unaided with an exercise tolerance of approximately 2 miles. There is no significant past medical history. On examination, the leg is externally rotated. Distal pulses are present and sensory and motor function is preserved. The injury is closed.

AP pelvis and lateral right hip X-rays are requested to assess for a fracture.

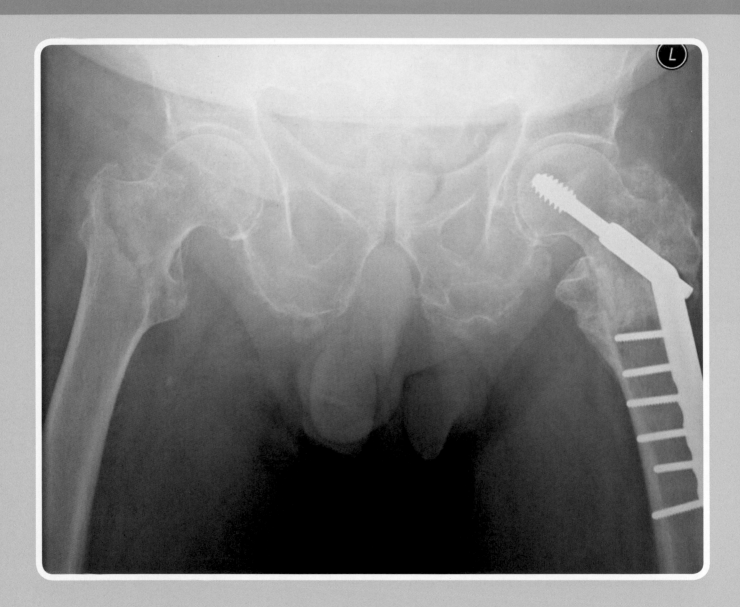

TECHNICAL INFORMATION

Patient ID: Anonymous.
Area: Pelvis.
Projection: AP.
Technical adequacy:

- Inadequate coverage – the entire pelvis is not included on the AP view. No lateral hip X-ray is available for review.
- Inadequate exposure – underexposed.
- The patient is not rotated.

● FRACTURE DETAILS

There is a fracture involving the right femoral neck in the intertrochanteric region.

The fracture is oblique, simple and extraarticular.

There is minimal displacement.

There is 5 degrees of varus angulation.

There is external rotation.

There is no shortening.

● JOINTS

There is no subluxation or dislocation.

There are no loose bodies.

There is no effusion or lipohaemarthrosis.

There are no arthritic changes.

● SOFT TISSUES

There is no soft tissue swelling.

There is no surgical emphysema.

● BACKGROUND BONE

There is a left long (>4 screws) dynamic hip screw and callus formation around the left femoral neck, in keeping with a previous healed fracture. The background bone is otherwise normal.

● BONE LESIONS

There is no bone lesion present.

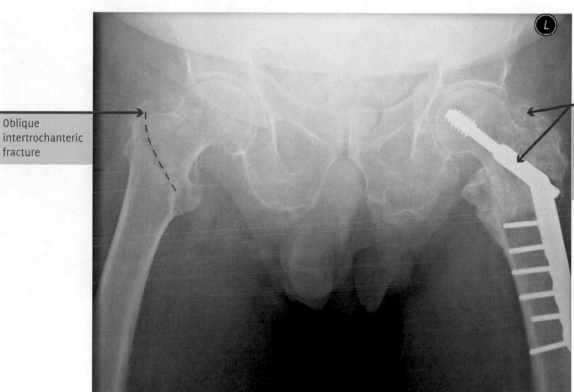

Oblique intertrochanteric fracture

Callus and dynamic hip screw related to old intertrochanteric fracture

SUMMARY AND DIFFERENTIAL

This X-ray demonstrates a minimally displaced right intertrochanteric neck of femur fracture.

INVESTIGATIONS AND MANAGEMENT

Appropriate analgesia should be provided.

The lateral right-hip X-ray should be reviewed to assess for fracture displacement or angulation and the AP X-ray should be repeated to include the entire pelvis.

The patient should be managed by a multidisciplinary team including orthogeriatricians who specialize in the management of hip fracture patients. As part of this treatment, a referral should be made to an orthopaedic surgeon for operative fixation with a dynamic hip screw.

A 55-year-old engineer fell off her bicycle. Subsequently, she was unable to mobilize and has presented to the ED. There is no significant past medical history. On examination, there is some mild pain on internal and external rotation of the left hip. There is no shortening. Distal pulses are present. Sensory and motor function is preserved. The injury is closed. Pain is improving, with limited mobilization now achievable.

AP pelvis and lateral left hip X-rays are requested to assess for a fracture.

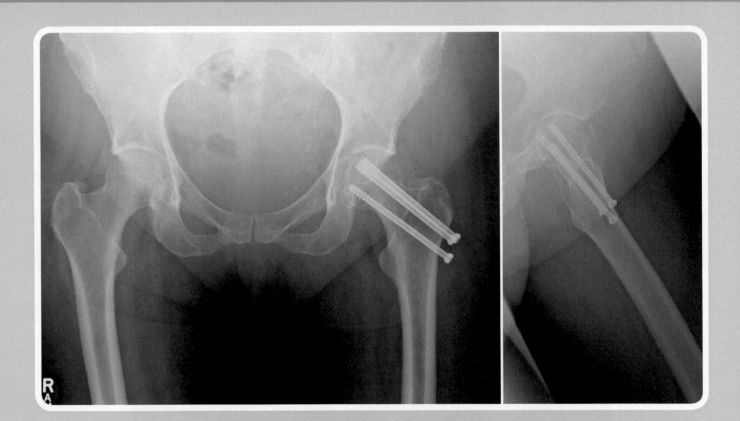

TECHNICAL INFORMATION

Patient ID: Anonymous.
Area: Left hip joint.
Projection: AP and lateral.
Technical adequacy:

- Adequate coverage.
- Adequate exposure.
- The patient is not rotated.

● FRACTURE DETAILS

There is no acute fracture.

● JOINTS

There is no subluxation or dislocation.

There are no loose bodies.

There is no effusion or lipohaemarthrosis.

There are arthritic changes present at both hip joints, namely decreased joint space and subchondral sclerosis.

● SOFT TISSUES

There is no soft tissue swelling.

There is no surgical emphysema.

● BACKGROUND BONE

There are left-sided cannulated hip screws in situ, indicative of a previous undisplaced intracapsular neck of femur fracture. There is no evidence of metalwork failure or fracture.

The background bone is normal.

● BONE LESIONS

There is no bone lesion present.

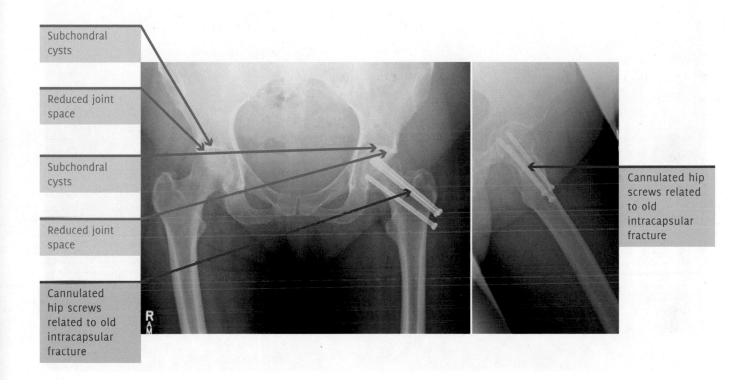

Subchondral cysts

Reduced joint space

Subchondral cysts

Reduced joint space

Cannulated hip screws related to old intracapsular fracture

Cannulated hip screws related to old intracapsular fracture

SUMMARY AND DIFFERENTIAL

These X-rays demonstrate no acute fracture on a background of bilateral osteoarthritic changes to the hips. Cannulated hip screws related to a previous left intracapsular neck of femur fracture are present.

INVESTIGATIONS AND MANAGEMENT

Appropriate analgesia should be provided.

Lifestyle modification including weight control and avoiding extra stress on weight-bearing joints should be provided.

GP follow-up should be provided if pain persists for consideration of further osteoarthritic management.

53

A 91-year-old female collapsed at home secondary to dizziness. She has been brought to the ED. She usually mobilizes with a stick. There is no significant past medical history. On examination, the patient is tender over the left hip. However, she is able to mobilize while fully weight-bearing on it and has a full range of hip movement. Distal pulses are present and sensory and motor function is preserved. The injury is closed.

AP pelvis and lateral left-hip X-rays are requested to assess for a fracture.

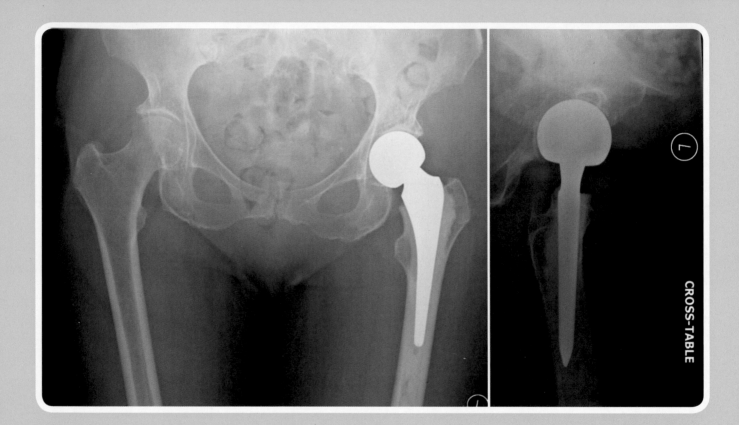

TECHNICAL INFORMATION

Patient ID: Anonymous.
Area: Left hip joint.
Projection: AP and lateral.
Technical adequacy:

- Adequate coverage.
- Adequate exposure.
- The patient is not rotated.

● FRACTURE DETAILS

There is no acute fracture.

● JOINTS

There is no subluxation or dislocation.

There are no loose bodies.

There is no effusion or lipohaemarthrosis.

There are no arthritic changes.

● SOFT TISSUES

There is no soft tissue swelling.

There is no surgical emphysema.

● BACKGROUND BONE

There is a cemented left-hip hemiarthroplasty, related to a previous intracapsular neck of femur fracture.

There is no evidence of metalwork failure/fracture or loosening.

The background bone is normal.

● BONE LESIONS

There is no bone lesion present.

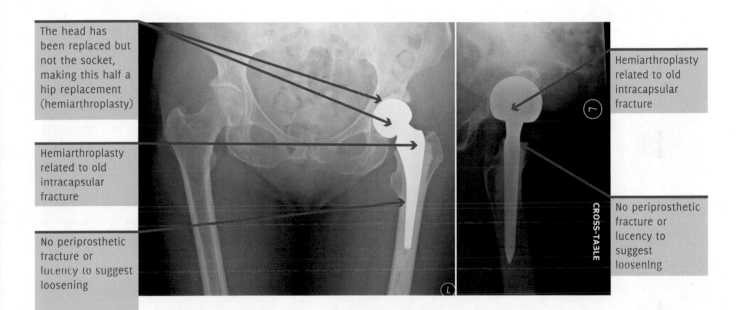

The head has been replaced but not the socket, making this half a hip replacement (hemiarthroplasty)

Hemiarthroplasty related to old intracapsular fracture

No periprosthetic fracture or lucency to suggest loosening

Hemiarthroplasty related to old intracapsular fracture

No periprosthetic fracture or lucency to suggest loosening

CROSS-TABLE

SUMMARY AND DIFFERENTIAL

These X-rays demonstrate no acute fracture. There is a left cemented hip hemiarthroplasty, without evidence of metalwork failure, periprosthetic fracture or loosening.

INVESTIGATIONS AND MANAGEMENT

Adequate analgesia should be provided.

No routine follow-up regarding the hip is required but the patient should be assessed in regards to her collapse.

A 94-year-old female, who is a nursing home resident with multiple comorbidities, was found on the floor by the nursing home staff. She has been brought to the ED by ambulance. She is normally only able to transfer from bed to chair. There is a past medical history of dementia and hypertension. On examination, the patient is tender over the left hip and there is bruising over the greater trochanter. The left leg is shortened by approximately 2 cm. The injury is closed, distal pulses are present and sensory and motor function is preserved.

AP pelvis and lateral left hip X-rays are requested to assess for a fracture.

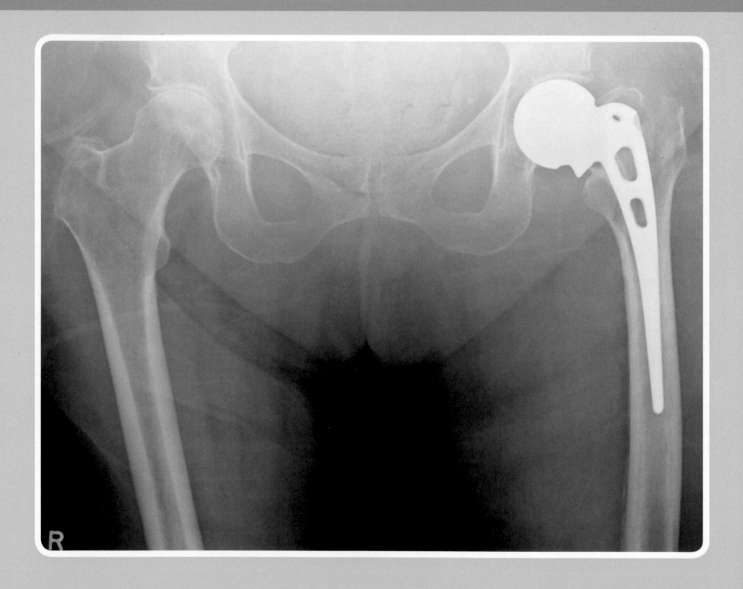

R

TECHNICAL INFORMATION

Patient ID: Anonymous.
Area: Left hip joint.
Projection: AP and lateral.
Technical adequacy:

- Inadequate coverage – the entire pelvis is not included on the AP view. No lateral hip X-ray is available for review.
- Adequate exposure.
- The patient is not rotated.

● FRACTURE DETAILS

There is a displaced fracture of the tip of the greater trochanter.

● JOINTS

There is no subluxation or dislocation.

There are no loose bodies.

There is no effusion or lipohaemarthrosis.

There are arthritic changes at the right hip joint, namely, loss of joint space and subchondral sclerosis.

● SOFT TISSUES

There is no soft tissue swelling.

There is no surgical emphysema.

● BACKGROUND BONE

There is an uncemented left-hip hemiarthroplasty, indicative of a previous intracapsular neck of femur fracture. There is no evidence of metalwork failure or fracture.

The background bone is osteopenic.

● BONE LESIONS

There is no bone lesion present.

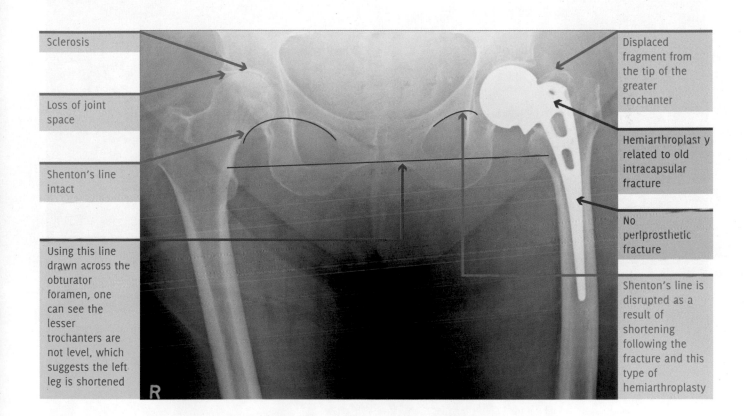

Sclerosis

Loss of joint space

Shenton's line intact

Using this line drawn across the obturator foramen, one can see the lesser trochanters are not level, which suggests the left leg is shortened

Displaced fragment from the tip of the greater trochanter

Hemiarthroplasty related to old intracapsular fracture

No periprosthetic fracture

Shenton's line is disrupted as a result of shortening following the fracture and this type of hemiarthroplasty

SUMMARY AND DIFFERENTIAL

This X-ray demonstrates no acute fracture. There is a left uncemented hip hemiarthroplasty without evidence of metalwork failure or periprosthetic fracture.

INVESTIGATIONS AND MANAGEMENT

Adequate analgesia should be provided.

The AP X-ray should be repeated to include the full pelvis and the lateral X-ray needs to be reviewed as well.

Osteopenia should be medically managed.

No routine orthopaedic follow-up is required.

A 12-year-old girl with obesity presents with 2-week history of pain in her left hip and groin associated with a limp. She has now become non-weight bearing on her left leg. She is systemically well. There is no significant past medical history. On examination, there is loss of active internal rotation, abduction and flexion of the left hip. On passive flexion of the hip, the leg externally rotates. She walks with an antalgic gait on the left.

An AP X-ray of the pelvis is requested to assess for fracture.

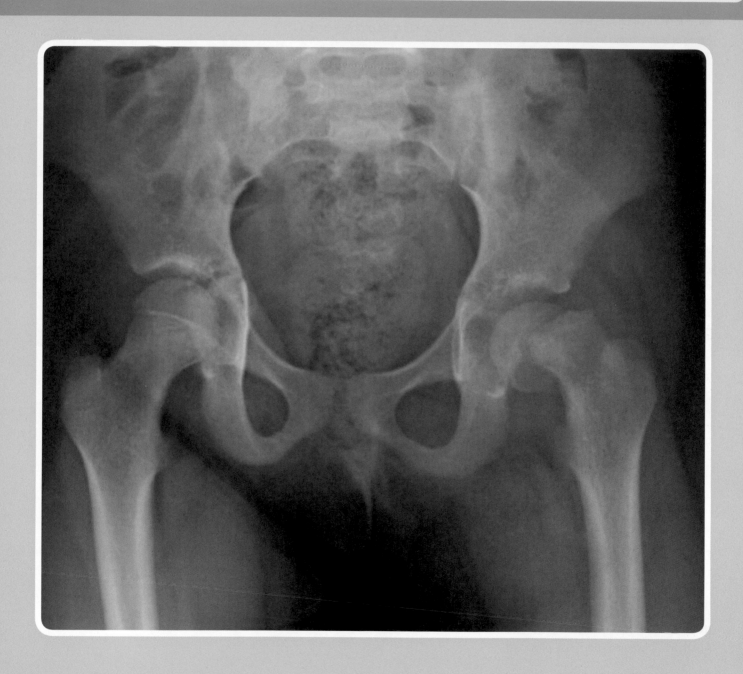

TECHNICAL INFORMATION

Patient ID: Anonymous.
Area: Pelvis.
Projection: AP.
Technical adequacy:

- Inadequate coverage as unable to visualize the superior aspects of the iliac bones.
- Adequate exposure.
- The patient is not rotated.

● FRACTURE DETAILS

There is a fracture of the left femoral neck, through the physis.

It is transverse, simple and extraarticular.

The distal fracture fragment is displaced superolaterally.

There is varus angulation.

There is external rotation.

There is shortening present.

● JOINTS

There is no subluxation or dislocation.

There are no loose bodies.

There is no effusion or lipohaemarthrosis.

There are no arthritic changes.

● SOFT TISSUES

There is no soft tissue swelling.

There is no surgical emphysema.

● BACKGROUND BONE

The background bone is normal.

● BONE LESIONS

There is no bone lesion present.

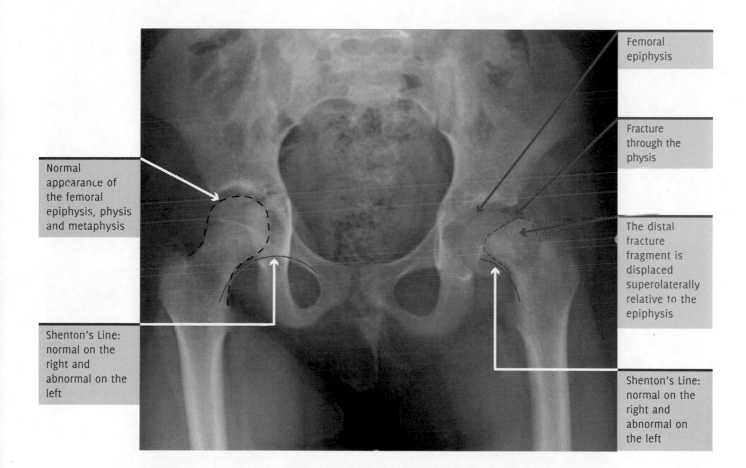

Normal appearance of the femoral epiphysis, physis and metaphysis

Shenton's Line: normal on the right and abnormal on the left

Femoral epiphysis

Fracture through the physis

The distal fracture fragment is displaced superolaterally relative to the epiphysis

Shenton's Line: normal on the right and abnormal on the left

SUMMARY AND DIFFERENTIAL

This X-ray demonstrates a displaced fracture through the physis of the left proximal femur. It is consistent with a left SUFE. This is consistent with a Salter-Harris Type 1 injury.

INVESTIGATIONS AND MANAGEMENT

Appropriate analgesia should be provided. A lateral X-ray of the hip is required.

An urgent referral should be made to an orthopaedic surgeon for further management. This may include percutaneous in situ fixation of the epiphysis with cannulated screws or open reduction and internal fixation. The choice of management is controversial.

There is also controversy regarding prophylactic fixation of the nonaffected side, but this could be considered.

A 12-year-old girl has been complaining for the last 2 weeks of pain in her right hip. This pain has been associated with sensations of hot and cold. There is no history of recent trauma. Her symptoms have not improved despite analgesia. Her GP has referred her for further investigation. There is no significant past medical history. On examination, the patient has a mild temperature of 37.7 °C, with a normal systemic examination: chest clear, heart sounds normal and abdomen soft and nontender. Examination of the hip elicits tenderness over the groin. There is no pain over the greater trochanter but there is pain on active internal and external rotation, as well as flexion, of the hip. The right lower limb is neurovascularly intact.

Frog-leg AP X-rays of the pelvis are requested to assess for a SUFE.

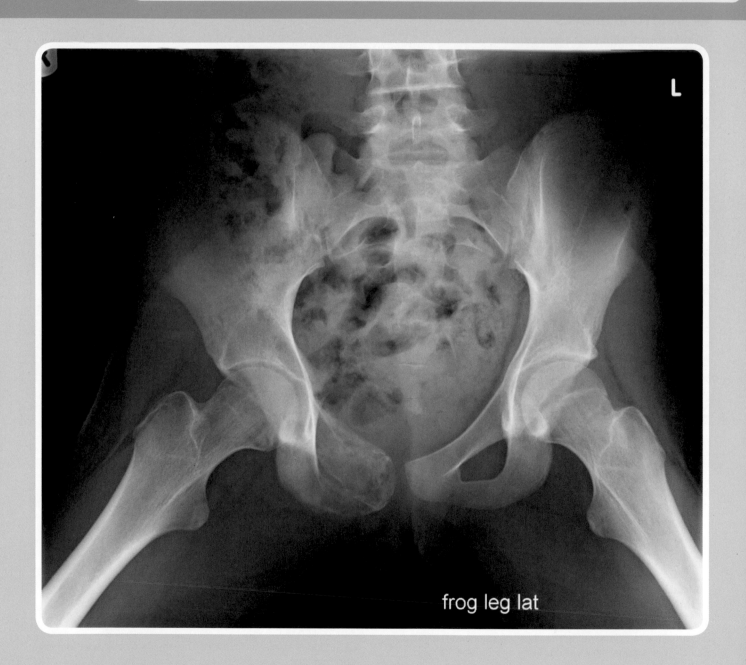

frog leg lat

TECHNICAL INFORMATION

Patient ID: Anonymous.
Area: Pelvis.
Projection: Frog-leg AP.
Technical adequacy:

- Adequate coverage.
- Adequate exposure.
- The patient is not rotated.

● FRACTURE DETAILS

There is no fracture.

● JOINTS

There is no subluxation or dislocation.

There are no loose bodies.

There is no effusion or lipohaemarthrosis.

There are no arthritic changes.

● SOFT TISSUES

There is soft tissue swelling in the right groin.

There is no surgical emphysema.

● BACKGROUND BONE

The background bone is normal.

● BONE LESIONS

There is a bone lesion present in the right pubic ramus.

It is lytic in appearance and expansile.

The zone of transition is wide.

There is evident bony destruction and periosteal reaction.

There is no soft tissue mass or component visible, although there is associated soft tissue swelling.

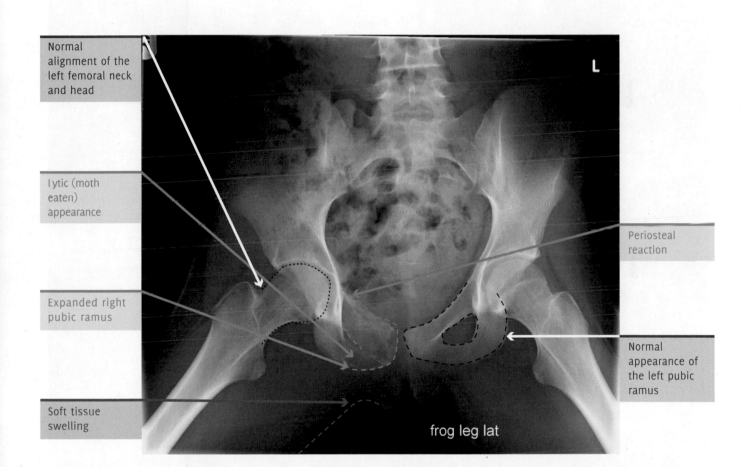

Normal alignment of the left femoral neck and head

lytic (moth eaten) appearance

Expanded right pubic ramus

Soft tissue swelling

Periosteal reaction

Normal appearance of the left pubic ramus

frog leg lat

SUMMARY AND DIFFERENTIAL

This X-ray demonstrates an aggressive and destructive bone lesion involving the right pubic ramus. Given its appearance, location and the age of the patient, the most likely cause is an Ewing's sarcoma. The differential also includes other primary tumours, such as osteosarcoma and metastases as well as osteomyelitis.

INVESTIGATIONS AND MANAGEMENT

Advice regarding analgesia should be provided.

Routine bloods, including a bone profile and inflammatory markers, should be taken.

An MRI should be requested to better define the lesion and for local staging.

A CT chest, abdomen and pelvis with IV contrast should be requested to stage the disease distally.

A referral should be made to a specialist in a bone tumour centre.

A 64-year-old secretary presents to her GP with a 7-week history of pain in her lower back that is exacerbated by movement. There is a history of weight loss over the last 2 months. On examination, there is a normal range of movement in the hips bilaterally. There is no evidence of radiculopathy. The patient is tender over the left iliac wing.

An AP X-ray of the pelvis is requested to assess for an insufficiency fracture or destructive lesion.

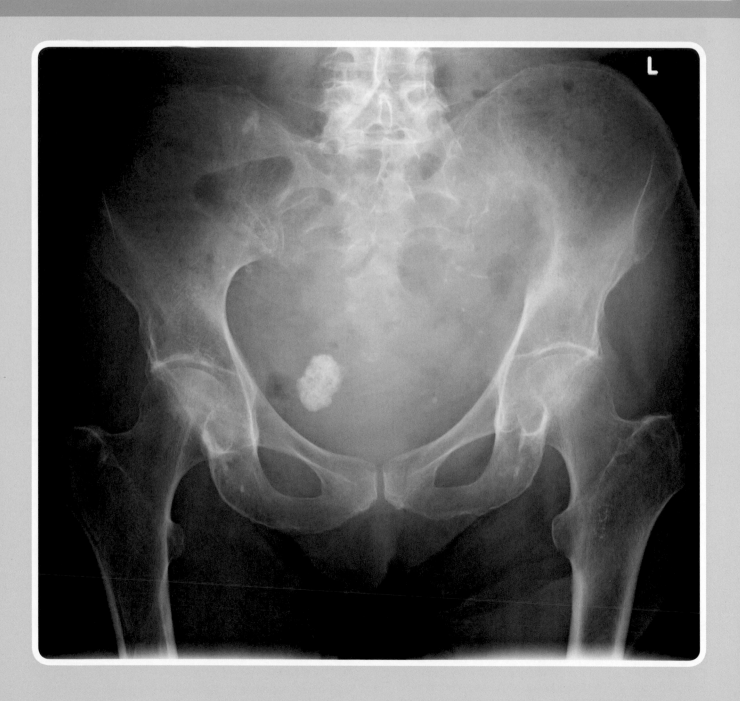

TECHNICAL INFORMATION

Patient ID: Anonymous.
Area: Pelvis.
Projection: AP.
Technical adequacy:

- Adequate coverage.
- Adequate exposure.
- The patient is not rotated.

● FRACTURE DETAILS

There is no fracture.

● JOINTS

There is no subluxation or dislocation.

There are no loose bodies.

There is no effusion or lipohaemarthrosis.

There are no arthritic changes.

● SOFT TISSUES

There is no soft tissue swelling.

There is no surgical emphysema.

There is a well-defined calcified mass projected over the right side of the pelvis. This is consistent with an incidental calcified fibroid.

● BACKGROUND BONE

The background bone is normal.

● BONE LESIONS

There is a bone lesion present in the left ilium.

It is lytic in appearance but not expansile.

The zone of transition is wide.

There is evident bony destruction, in particular involving the pelvic brim on the left.

There is no periosteal reaction.

A soft tissue mass or component is suspected in the left side of the pelvis.

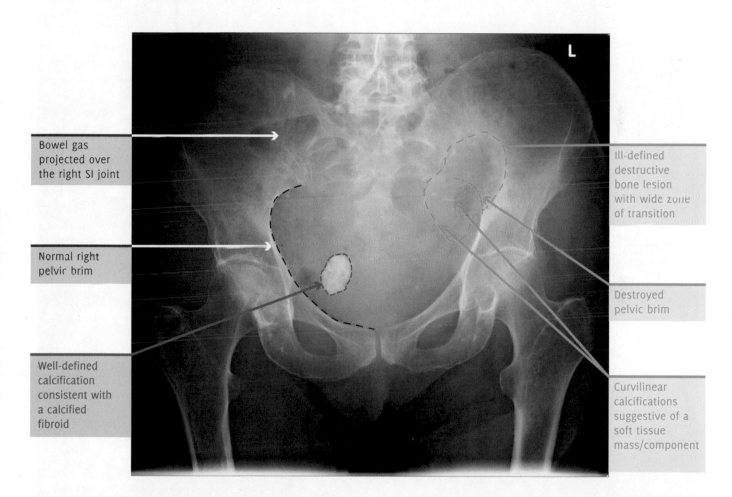

Bowel gas projected over the right SI joint

Normal right pelvic brim

Well-defined calcification consistent with a calcified fibroid

Ill-defined destructive bone lesion with wide zone of transition

Destroyed pelvic brim

Curvilinear calcifications suggestive of a soft tissue mass/component

SUMMARY AND DIFFERENTIAL

This X-ray demonstrates an aggressive bone lesion in the left ilium, causing bony destruction. The most likely differential diagnosis in a patient of this age is a metastatic deposit. The primary is likely to be either a lung or breast cancer, as these are the most common types. Less likely is a primary bone tumour such as osteosarcoma.

INVESTIGATIONS AND MANAGEMENT

The patient requires further investigation. The disease should be staged locally with an MRI and distally with a CT scan of the chest, abdomen and pelvis with contrast and a bone scan. Blood tests including a myeloma screen should be sent and liaison with an oncology team is advised before requesting tumour markers.

Treatment depends on the cause of the lytic bony lesion but if this is metastatic disease then chemotherapy, radiotherapy or tumour specific therapies such as trastuzumab (Herceptin) for breast cancer would form the basis for treatment.

A 74-year-old partially blind woman fell over her granddaughter's toy doll that was left on the floor. She landed on her left side and was found on the floor. She has since been unable to mobilize and has been brought into the ED by ambulance. There is no significant past medical history. On examination, there is bruising around the left hip with pain on palpation over the greater trochanter and in the groin. All movements of the hip are very painful. Distal pulses are present and sensory and motor function is preserved. The injury is closed.

AP and lateral X-rays of the pelvis and left hip are requested to assess for a fracture.

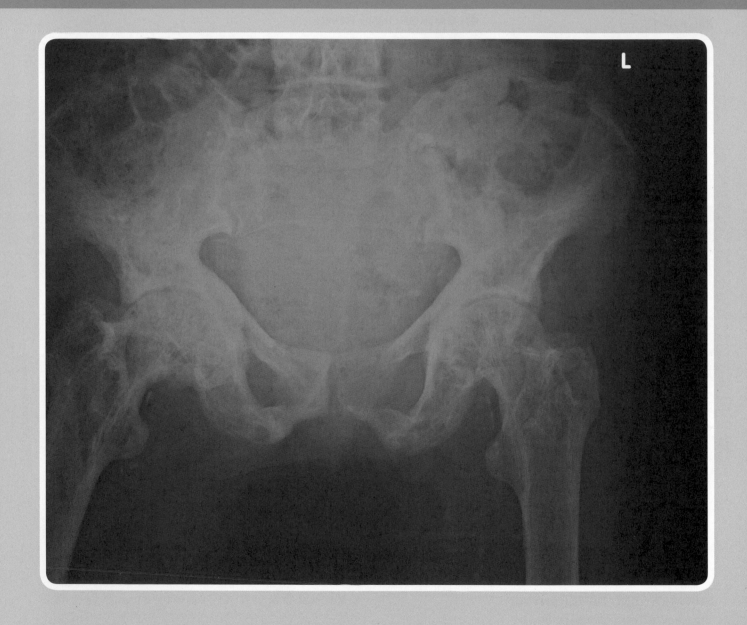

L

TECHNICAL INFORMATION

Patient ID: Anonymous.
Area: AP pelvis and lateral hip.
Projection: AP and lateral.
Technical adequacy:

- Inadequate coverage – only the AP view is available for review.
- Adequate exposure.
- The patient is not rotated.

● FRACTURE DETAILS

There is a fracture involving the intertrochanteric region of the left femoral neck.

The fracture is oblique, simple and extraarticular.

There is no displacement.

There is no angulation.

There is no rotation.

There is no shortening.

● JOINTS

There is no subluxation or dislocation.

There are no loose bodies.

There is no effusion or lipohaemarthrosis.

There are arthritic changes in both hips. This is more marked on the right where there is osteophyte formation and almost complete loss of joint space. Given the background bone abnormality, it is difficult to assess for subchondral sclerosis and cyst formation.

● SOFT TISSUES

There is no soft tissue swelling.

There is no surgical emphysema.

Vascular calcification of the femoral vessels is present.

● BACKGROUND BONE

The background bone of the pelvis and proximal femur is abnormal.

There is cortical and trabecular thickening and sclerosis, in particular involving the iliopectinal and ilioischial lines on the right. There is bony expansion.

● BONE LESIONS

There is no focal bone lesion present.

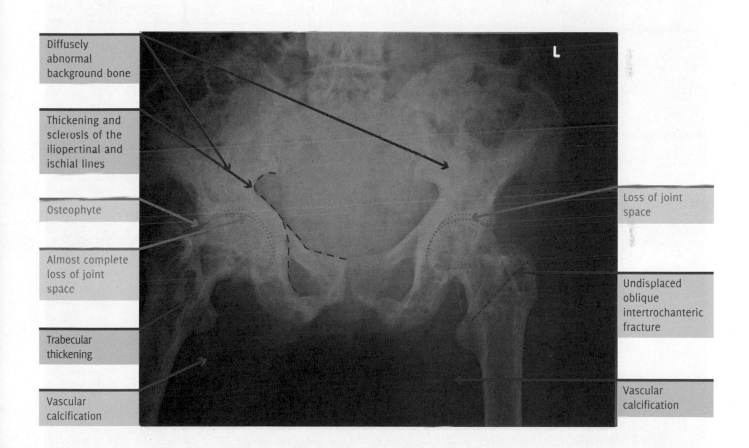

Diffusely abnormal background bone

Thickening and sclerosis of the iliopectinal and ischial lines

Osteophyte

Almost complete loss of joint space

Trabecular thickening

Vascular calcification

Loss of joint space

Undisplaced oblique intertrochanteric fracture

Vascular calcification

SUMMARY AND DIFFERENTIAL

This X-ray demonstrates an undisplaced left intertrochanteric femoral neck fracture. There is a diffuse background bone abnormality, which particularly affects the pelvis and is consistent with Paget's disease.

INVESTIGATIONS AND MANAGEMENT

Advice regarding analgesia should be provided.

A lateral X-ray is required.

The patient should be managed by a multidisciplinary team including orthogeriatricians who specialize in the management of hip fracture patients. The patient should be cared for with a standardized care pathway. Input is required from orthopaedics for surgical management, which will likely be with a dynamic hip screw.

A 52-year-old woman presents having fallen down 10 steps at a garden centre. She fell onto her left side and is now complaining of pain. She is no longer able to weight bear on the left side. She has a history of pelvic malignancy and right-sided hydronephrosis. On examination, the left leg is shortened and externally rotated. Axial loading of the hip is painful, and the patient is unable to mobilize. Distal pulses are present and sensory and motor function is preserved. The injury is closed.

An AP X-ray of the pelvis is requested to assess for fracture.

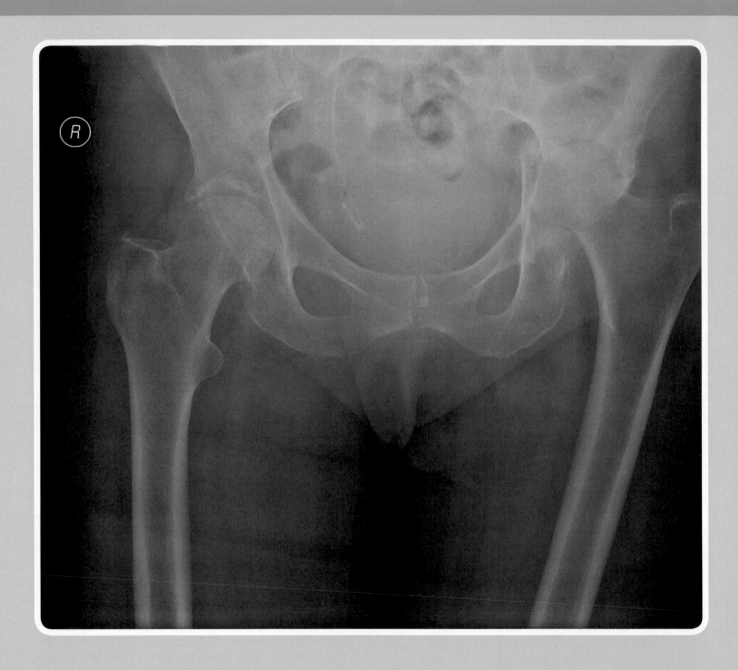

TECHNICAL INFORMATION

Patient ID: Anonymous.
Area: Pelvis.
Projection: AP.
Technical adequacy:

- Inadequate coverage, as the proximal part of the pelvis is not completely imaged.
- Adequate exposure.
- The patient is not rotated.

● FRACTURE DETAILS

There is a fracture involving the left acetabulum.

The fracture is intraarticular.

There is medial and superior displacement of the left femoral head (acetabular protrusion).

There is no angulation.

There is no rotation.

There is shortening.

● JOINTS

There is no subluxation or dislocation.

There are no loose bodies.

There is no effusion or lipohaemarthrosis.

There are no arthritic changes.

● SOFT TISSUES

There is no soft tissue swelling.

There is no surgical emphysema.

Appearance of a partially imaged linear structure is seen descending in the right side of the pelvis. Its location and appearance are in keeping with that of a ureteric stent.

● BACKGROUND BONE

The background bone is normal.

● BONE LESIONS

There is no bone lesion present.

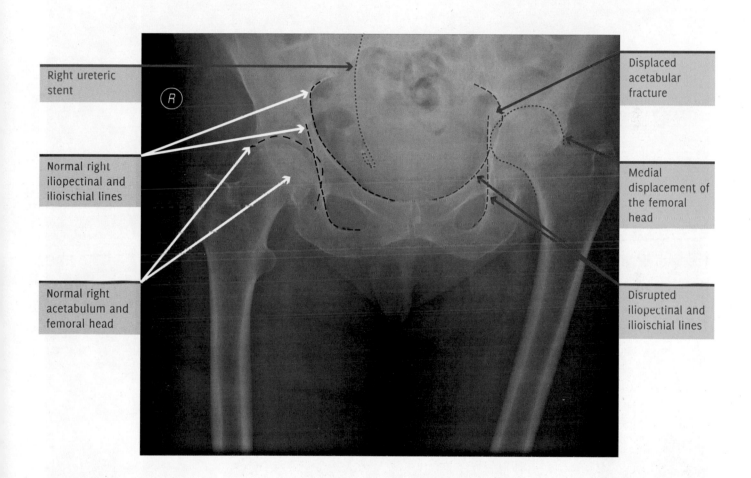

Right ureteric stent

Normal right iliopectinal and ilioischial lines

Normal right acetabulum and femoral head

Displaced acetabular fracture

Medial displacement of the femoral head

Disrupted iliopectinal and ilioischial lines

SUMMARY AND DIFFERENTIAL

This X-ray demonstrates a left acetabular fracture, with medial and superior displacement of the acetabulum and femoral head.

INVESTIGATIONS AND MANAGEMENT

Advice regarding analgesia should be provided.

The patient should be referred for further imaging in the form of Judet views and a CT scan. A referral is required to orthopaedics who may consider surgery depending on the extent of underlying malignancy, life expectancy and severity of the fracture.

A 15-year-old girl was a passenger in a road traffic collision. She has been brought to the ED via ambulance to a major paediatric trauma centre. She has a pelvic binder in situ. Following a primary survey, the patient is stable, and an isolated pelvic injury is suspected. There is no significant past medical history. On examination, she is tender over the sacrum and in the groin. Range of movement at the hip is painful but not limited. Distal pulses and motor and sensory function is preserved. The injury is closed.

AP X-rays of the pelvis are requested to assess for a fracture.

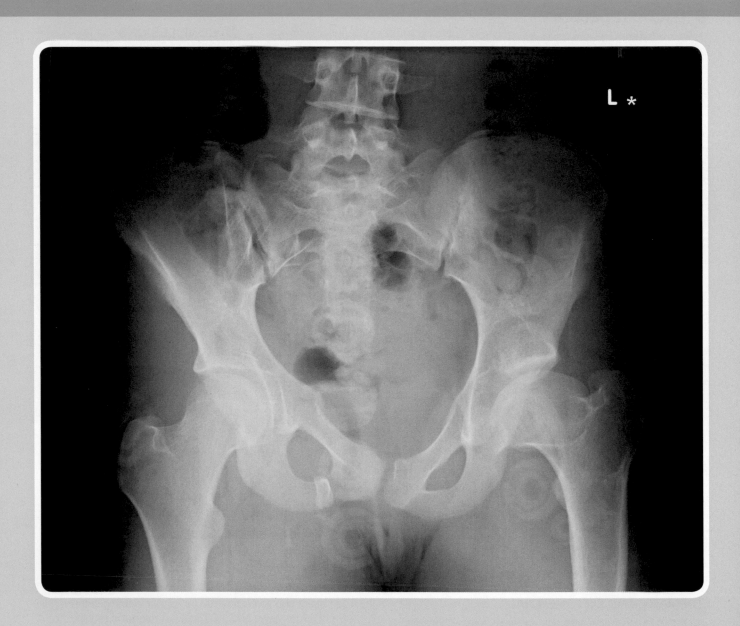

TECHNICAL INFORMATION

Patient ID: Anonymous.
Area: Pelvis.
Projection: AP.
Technical adequacy:

- Adequate coverage.
- Adequate exposure.
- The patient is not rotated.

● FRACTURE DETAILS

There are fractures involving the right superior and inferior pubic rami.

The fractures are longitudinal, simple and extraarticular.

There is displacement of the pubic rami fractures.

There is no angulation.

There is no rotation.

There is no shortening.

There is a fracture involving the right sacral alar.

The fracture is longitudinal and simple. It appears to involve the right sacro-iliac joint, which is widened.

There is no displacement.

There is no angulation.

There is no rotation.

There is no shortening.

There is an undisplaced fracture involving one of the lower right anterior sacral foramina.

There is no angulation.

There is no rotation.

There is no shortening.

● JOINTS

The right sacro-iliac joint appears widened distally, suggesting partial disruption.

The left sacro-iliac joint and pubic symphysis appear intact.

There are no loose bodies.

There is no effusion or lipohaemarthrosis.

The left femoral head and neck is dysplastic and there is an abnormal configuration. This may relate to previous developmental dysplasia of the hip, a slipped upper femoral epiphysis or Perthes disease.

● SOFT TISSUES

There is no soft tissue swelling.

There is no surgical emphysema.

There is a pelvic binder in situ.

● BACKGROUND BONE

The background bone is normal.

● BONE LESIONS

There is no bone lesion present.

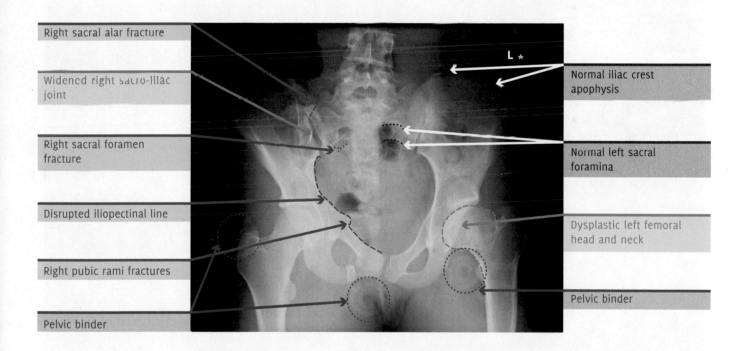

Right sacral alar fracture

Widened right sacro-iliac joint

Right sacral foramen fracture

Disrupted iliopectinal line

Right pubic rami fractures

Pelvic binder

L *

Normal iliac crest apophysis

Normal left sacral foramina

Dysplastic left femoral head and neck

Pelvic binder

SUMMARY AND DIFFERENTIAL

This X-ray demonstrates a right superior and inferior pubic rami fracture. There is also a right sacral alar fracture and widening of the right sacro-iliac joint. An undisplaced right anterior sacral foramen fracture can also be seen. These injuries represent a significant pelvic injury.

INVESTIGATIONS AND MANAGEMENT

Advice regarding analgesia should be provided.

The patient should be managed using the ATLS guidelines to assess for further injuries.

The patient should have an urgent CT of the pelvis and the sacrum with IV contrast. This is needed to further characterize the bony injuries and assess for soft tissue or visceral injuries, in particular a traumatic bladder injury.

The case should be discussed with the paediatric orthopaedic and pelvic surgeons who will consider possible surgical intervention.

A 55-year-old woman who suffers from rheumatoid arthritis presents with several months of worsening right hip pain. This has progressed to the point where she is now struggling to weight bear. There is a past medical history of significant rheumatoid arthritis in both hands. This has previously been treated with corticosteroids. On examination, the right hip is painful and there is limited movement in all directions. The patient has an antalgic gait on the right when mobilizing.

An AP X-ray of the pelvis is requested to assess for degenerative changes.

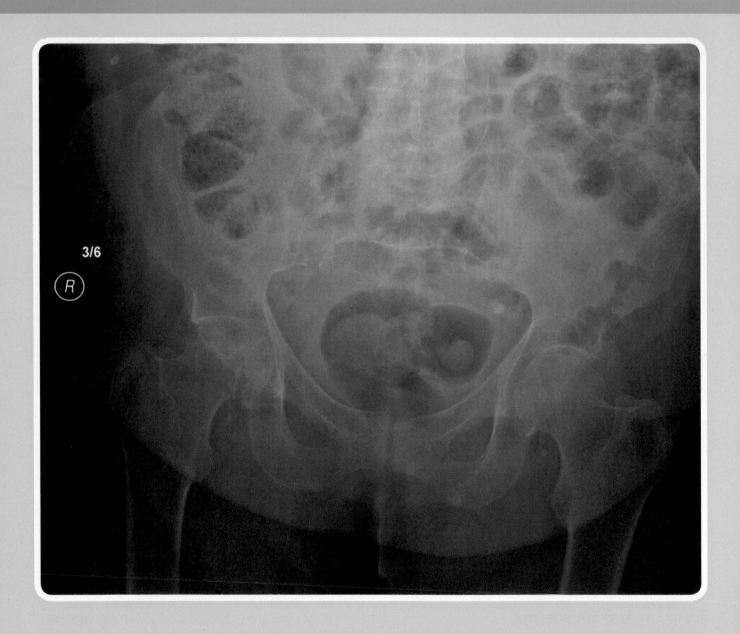

TECHNICAL INFORMATION

Patient ID: Anonymous.
Area: Pelvis.
Projection: AP.
Technical adequacy:

- Adequate coverage.
- Adequate exposure.
- The patient is not rotated.

● FRACTURE DETAILS

There is no acute fracture.

● JOINTS

There is no subluxation or dislocation.

There are no loose bodies.

There is no effusion or lipohaemarthrosis.

There is femoral head collapse with secondary arthritis of the right hip.

The left hip shows signs of arthritis with loss of joint space but without femoral head collapse.

● SOFT TISSUES

There is no soft tissue swelling.

There is no surgical emphysema.

Vascular calcifications are present in the femoral vessels.

Calcification markings are projected over the lower lumbar spine.

● BACKGROUND BONE

The background bone is normal.

● BONE LESIONS

There is no bone lesion present.

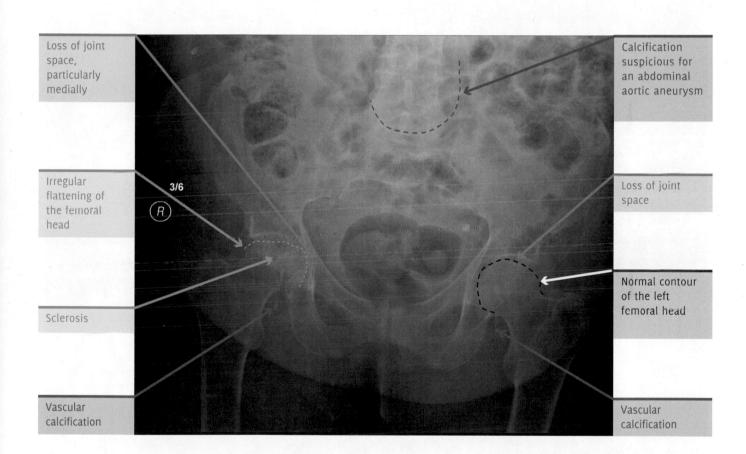

Loss of joint space, particularly medially

Irregular flattening of the femoral head

3/6

R

Sclerosis

Vascular calcification

Calcification suspicious for an abdominal aortic aneurysm

Loss of joint space

Normal contour of the left femoral head

Vascular calcification

SUMMARY AND DIFFERENTIAL

This X-ray demonstrates features consistent with avascular necrosis of the right femoral head. This may be related to previous steroid use although the most common cause of AVN is idiopathic. There is flattening of the femoral head and joint space narrowing.

The calcified region projected over the lower lumbar spine is suspicious for a calcified abdominal aortic aneurysm.

INVESTIGATIONS AND MANAGEMENT

Advice regarding analgesia should be provided.

A referral should be made to an orthopaedic surgeon who may consider a total hip arthroplasty.

An abdominal ultrasound scan should be requested to further assess the potential abdominal aortic aneurysm.

An 89-year-old woman had an unwitnessed fall in the middle of the night. She lives in a care home and is brought to the ED by one of the staff. She is unable to weight bear. She has a history of cognitive impairment. On examination, there is pain over the groin on palpation and on flexion of the right hip. Range of movement in the right hip is normal. Distal pulses are present and sensory and motor function is preserved. The injury is closed.

An AP X-ray of the pelvis is requested to assess for a fracture.

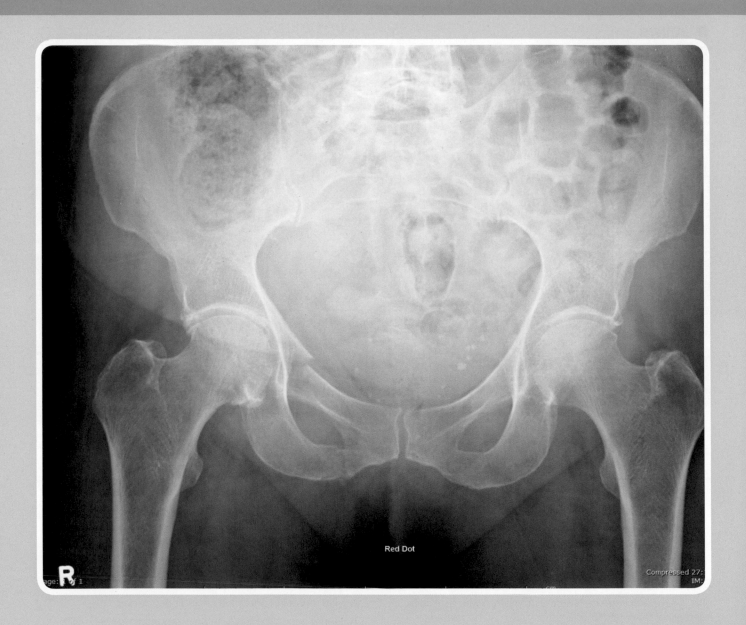

Red Dot

TECHNICAL INFORMATION

Patient ID: Anonymous.
Area: Pelvis.
Projection: AP.
Technical adequacy:

- Adequate coverage.
- Adequate exposure.
- The patient is not rotated.

● FRACTURE DETAILS

There are fractures involving the right superior and inferior pubic rami.

The fractures are longitudinal, simple and extraarticular.

Both are minimally displaced.

There is no angulation.

There is no rotation.

There is no shortening.

● JOINTS

There is no subluxation or dislocation.

There are no loose bodies.

There is no effusion or lipohaemarthrosis.

There are arthritic changes in both hip joints. In particular, there is loss of joint space, subchondral sclerosis and osteophyte formation.

● SOFT TISSUES

There is no soft tissue swelling.

There is no surgical emphysema.

Minor calcification of the left femoral vessels is present.

● BACKGROUND BONE

The background bone is normal.

● BONE LESIONS

There is no bone lesion present.

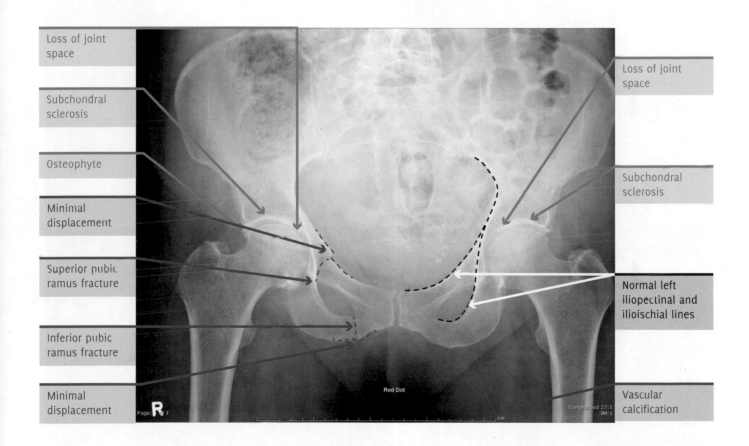

Loss of joint space

Subchondral sclerosis

Osteophyte

Minimal displacement

Superior pubic ramus fracture

Inferior pubic ramus fracture

Minimal displacement

Loss of joint space

Subchondral sclerosis

Normal left iliopectinal and ilioischial lines

Vascular calcification

Red Dot

SUMMARY AND DIFFERENTIAL

This X-ray demonstrates right superior and inferior pubic rami fractures.

INVESTIGATIONS AND MANAGEMENT

Advice regarding analgesia should be provided.

The patient should be managed nonoperatively with physiotherapy and weight bearing as tolerated.

A 55-year-old woman presents to the ED with pain following a fall onto her left hip. There is a 3-month history of left hip pain and weight loss. On examination, the leg is shortened and externally rotated. Any movement, especially internal and external rotation in an extended position, is painful. Distal pulses are present and sensory and motor function is preserved. The injury is closed.

AP and lateral X-rays of the left hip are requested to assess for fracture.

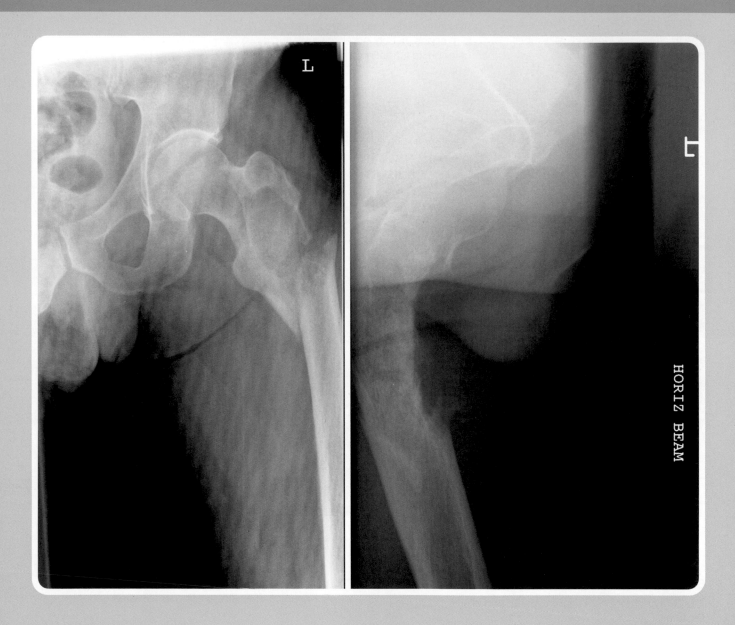

TECHNICAL INFORMATION

Patient ID: Anonymous.
Area: Left hip.
Projection: AP and lateral.
Technical adequacy:

- The posterior aspect of the proximal femur has not been fully included on the lateral X-ray.
- Adequate exposure.
- The patient is not rotated.

FRACTURE DETAILS

There is a fracture involving the proximal femur.

The fracture is oblique, simple and extraarticular.

There is mild lateral displacement.

There is medial angulation.

There is no rotation.

There is shortening.

JOINTS

There is no subluxation or dislocation.

There are no loose bodies.

There is no effusion or lipohaemarthrosis.

There are no arthritic changes.

SOFT TISSUES

There is no soft tissue swelling.

There is no surgical emphysema.

BACKGROUND BONE

The background bone is normal.

BONE LESIONS

There is a bone lesion present in the proximal femur.

It is lytic in appearance.

It is not expansile.

The zone of transition is mixed, appearing narrow in places and wide in others.

There is bony destruction present.

There is no periosteal reaction.

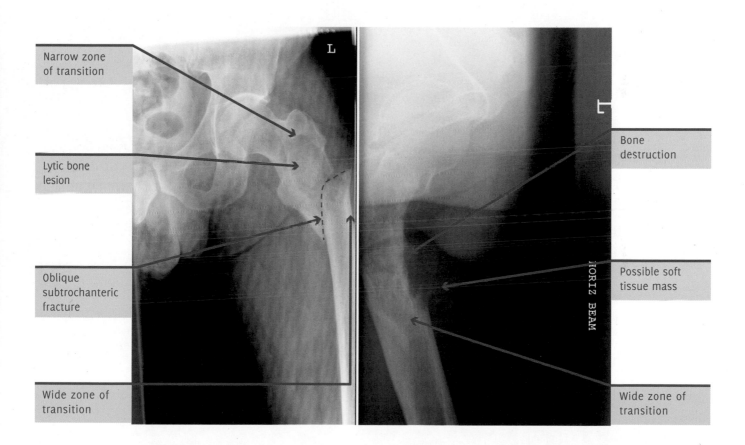

Narrow zone of transition

Lytic bone lesion

Oblique subtrochanteric fracture

Wide zone of transition

Bone destruction

Possible soft tissue mass

Wide zone of transition

SUMMARY AND DIFFERENTIAL

Both X-rays demonstrate a displaced subtrochanteric fracture associated with an aggressive appearing bone lesion in the proximal femur.

Given the age of the patient, the injury pattern most likely represents a pathological fracture of a bony metastasis although a primary bone tumour is also a possibility.

INVESTIGATIONS AND MANAGEMENT

Appropriate analgesia should be provided.

The bone lesion needs to be staged locally and distally.

A CT of the chest, abdomen and pelvis with IV contrast should be requested to attempt to identify a primary tumour and for staging.

A full-length femoral X-ray should be requested to assess for further lesions.

A referral should be made to an oncology team for a new diagnosis of malignancy and to an orthopaedic surgeon who may consider femoral intramedullary nailing.

The patient can immediately fully weight bear following femoral intramedullary nailing.

A 20-year-old man presents with increasing thigh pain and swelling over the past 3 months. There is no history of trauma. There is no significant past medical history. On examination, there is a 20×10 cm fixed, firm swelling over the anterior thigh, with tenderness on palpation.

AP and lateral X-rays of the left femur are requested to assess for bony destruction.

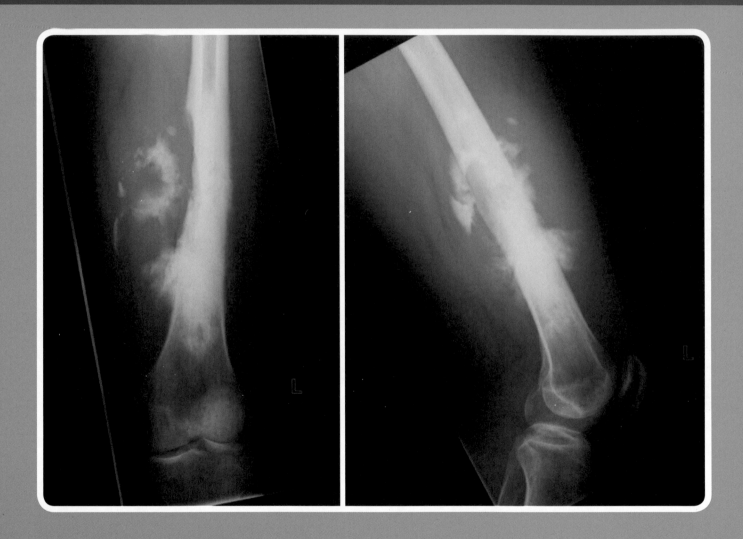

TECHNICAL INFORMATION

Patient ID: Anonymous.
Area: Left femur.
Projection: AP/lateral.
Technical adequacy:

- Adequate coverage.
- Adequate exposure.
- The patient is not rotated.

● FRACTURE DETAILS

There is no fracture.

● JOINTS

There is no subluxation or dislocation.

There are no loose bodies.

There is no effusion or lipohaemarthrosis.

There are no arthritic changes.

● SOFT TISSUES

There is a large soft tissue mass, which is partly ossified, and infiltrates into the bone. It is most prominent medial to the mid-femur.

There is no surgical emphysema.

● BACKGROUND BONE

The background bone is normal.

● BONE LESIONS

There is a bone lesion present in the diaphysis of the femur.

It is sclerotic.

It is expansile.

The zone of transition is wide, and its margins are poorly demarcated.

There is medullary and cortical bony destruction.

There is periosteal reaction, which has a sunburst appearance.

There is a partially ossified soft tissue component medially.

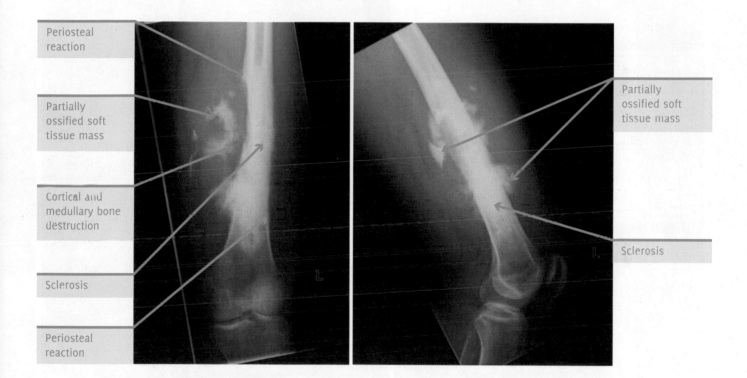

Periosteal reaction

Partially ossified soft tissue mass

Cortical and medullary bone destruction

Sclerosis

Periosteal reaction

Partially ossified soft tissue mass

Sclerosis

SUMMARY AND DIFFERENTIAL

These X-rays demonstrate a destructive femoral bone lesion with periosteal reaction and a soft tissue component. This description is in keeping with an aggressive bone lesion. Given the age of the patient and location of the lesion, it is most likely an osteosarcoma. Other differentials to consider include Ewing sarcoma and metastases.

INVESTIGATIONS AND MANAGEMENT

The lesion needs to be staged both locally and distally. Local staging is achieved with an MRI of the femur.

A CT of the chest, abdomen and pelvis with IV contrast should be requested to stage distally.

The patient should be referred to a specialist tumour centre for biopsy and definitive management. Options may include distal femoral replacement or limb amputation. Any bony or soft tissue lesion where there is any doubt about its nature should be referred to a specialist tumour centre for an opinion.

A 68-year-old man presents to the ED with severe pain in his right thigh after a fall from standing height. His past medical history is significant for type II diabetes and hypertension. On examination, the patient is tender over the mid-thigh and there is an obvious deformity. Distal pulses are present and sensory and motor function is preserved. The injury is closed.

AP and lateral X-rays of the right femur are requested to assess for fracture.

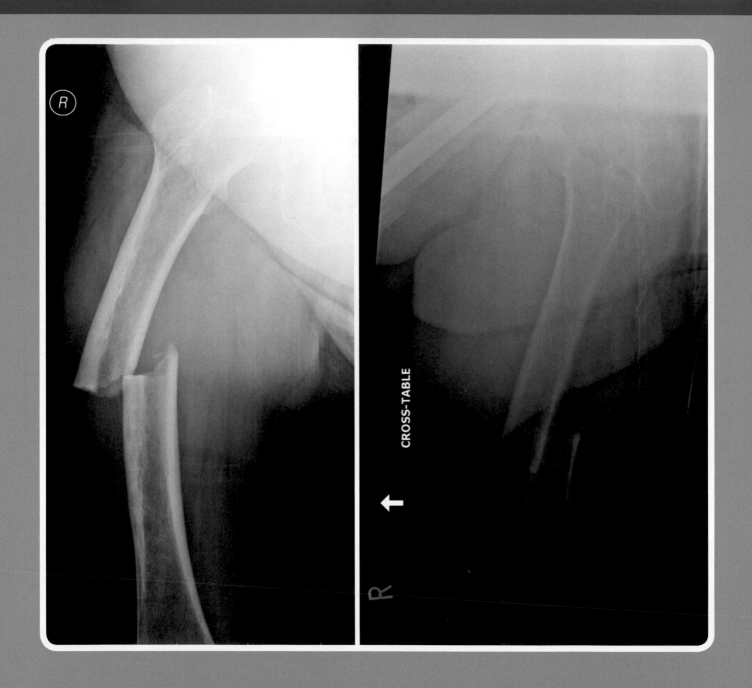

CROSS-TABLE

R

TECHNICAL INFORMATION

Patient ID: Anonymous.
Area: Right femur.
Projection: AP and lateral.
Technical adequacy:

- Adequate coverage.
- Adequate exposure.
- The patient is not rotated.

● FRACTURE DETAILS

There is a fracture of the middle third of the femur.

The fracture is transverse, comminuted and extraarticular.

There is posterior and medial displacement.

There is medial angulation.

There is no rotation.

There is shortening of the femur.

● JOINTS

The hip joint is not formally visualized.

However, there is no subluxation or dislocation.

There are no loose bodies.

There is no effusion or lipohaemarthrosis.

There are no arthritic changes.

● SOFT TISSUES

There is soft tissue swelling as expected with a femoral fracture.

There is no surgical emphysema.

● BACKGROUND BONE

The background bone is normal.

● BONE LESIONS

There is no bony lesion present.

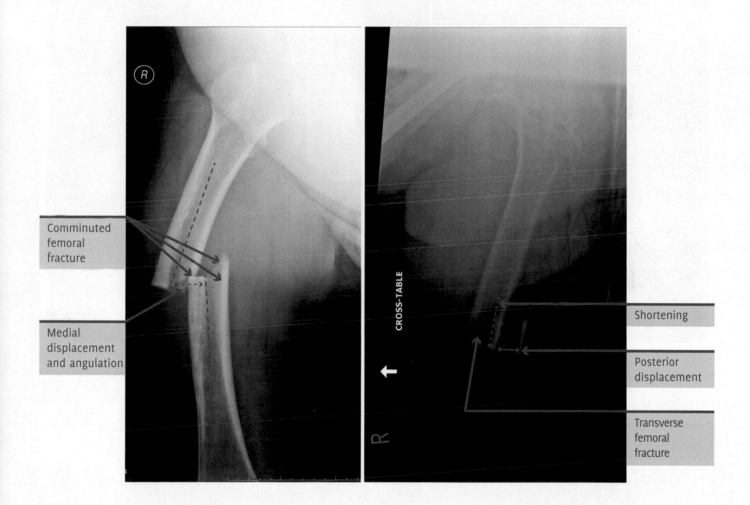

Comminuted femoral fracture

Medial displacement and angulation

CROSS-TABLE

Shortening

Posterior displacement

Transverse femoral fracture

SUMMARY AND DIFFERENTIAL

Both X-rays demonstrate a transverse midshaft fracture of the femur.

INVESTIGATIONS AND MANAGEMENT

Appropriate analgesia should be provided.

Skin traction should be applied to allow good pain relief.

X-rays of the whole femur are required to exclude metastatic bone disease.

A referral should be made to an orthopaedic surgeon.

The patient will most likely be treated with intramedullary nail fixation.

A 66-year-old woman has been brought to the local trauma unit as a trauma call. She fell down five steps at a train station. She felt her knee 'go out to the side' as she fell. Following an ATLS assessment with no significant findings on primary survey, she is found to have severe knee pain and states that she is unable to straighten or stand on her leg. There is no significant past medical history. On examination, the patient is tender over the joint line of the left knee with a moderate effusion. All movements are painful. Proper assessment of the ligaments is impossible because of pain. Distal pulses are present, sensory and motor function is preserved and compartments are soft. The injury is closed.

AP and lateral X-rays of the left knee are requested to assess for a fracture.

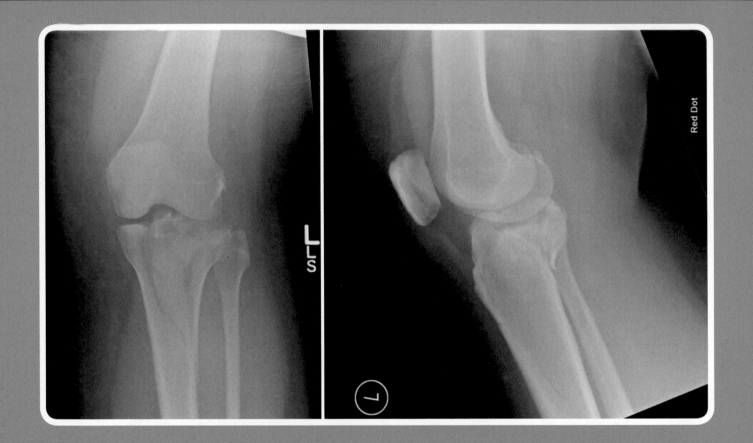

TECHNICAL INFORMATION

Patient ID: Anonymous.
Area: Left knee.
Projection: AP and lateral.
Technical adequacy:

- Adequate coverage.
- Adequate exposure.
- The patient is not rotated.

● FRACTURE DETAILS

There is a fracture involving the plateau of the tibia, with a split extending proximally from the medial plateau to the lateral cortex.

The fracture is comminuted and intraarticular.

There is displacement with depression of the lateral tibial articular surface of at least 5 mm.

There is no angulation.

There is no rotation.

There is no shortening.

● JOINTS

There is no subluxation or dislocation.

There are no loose bodies.

A knee joint effusion with a fat fluid level is present, indicating a lipohaemarthrosis.

There are no arthritic changes.

● SOFT TISSUES

There is soft tissue swelling around the knee joint.

There is no surgical emphysema.

● BACKGROUND BONE

The background bone is normal.

● BONE LESIONS

There is no bone lesion present.

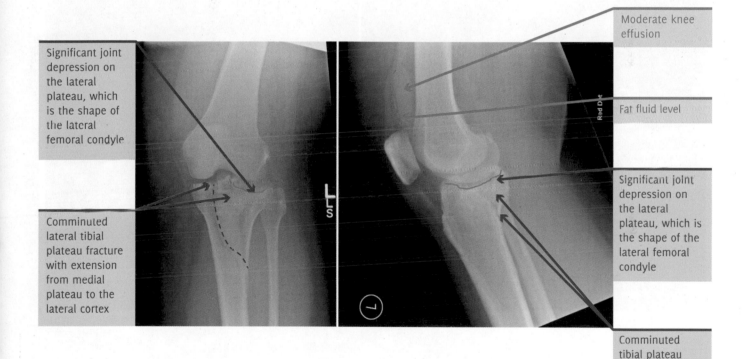

Significant joint depression on the lateral plateau, which is the shape of the lateral femoral condyle

Comminuted lateral tibial plateau fracture with extension from medial plateau to the lateral cortex

Moderate knee effusion

Fat fluid level

Significant joint depression on the lateral plateau, which is the shape of the lateral femoral condyle

Comminuted tibial plateau fracture

SUMMARY AND DIFFERENTIAL

Both X-rays demonstrate a left tibial plateau fracture with lipohaemarthrosis. The injury has been caused by a valgus force where the lateral femoral condyle has been driven into the lateral tibial plateau. This is therefore a Schatzker type 2 fracture.

INVESTIGATIONS AND MANAGEMENT

Advice regarding analgesia should be provided. An above knee back slab should be applied for pain relief.

A CT scan should be undertaken to further delineate the fracture pattern and degree of comminution.

A referral should be made to an orthopaedic surgeon for surgical fixation.

A 56-year-old male has been brought to the ED by ambulance. He slipped whilst descending a ladder, trapping his right foot between two rungs, and consequently twisting his leg. When this happened, he felt a snap and had instant pain in the right leg. There is no significant past medical history. On examination, there is a visibly deformed right leg, with swelling and tenderness over the distal tibia. There is also tenderness to palpation over the proximal fibula. Distal pulses are present and sensory and motor function is preserved. The injury is closed.

AP and lateral X-rays of the right leg are requested to assess for a fracture.

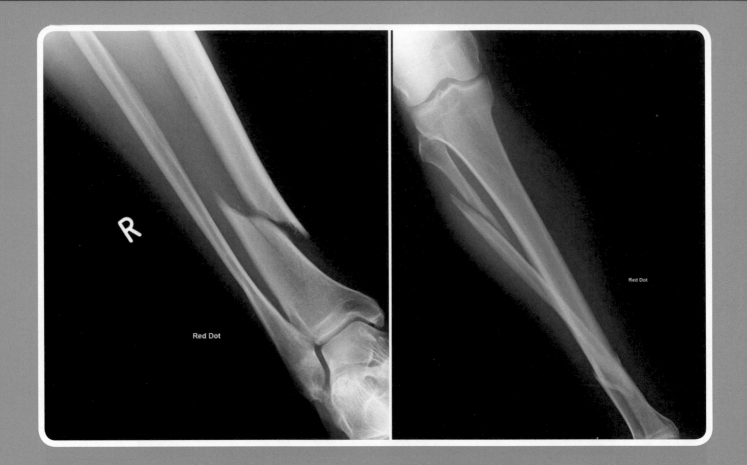

TECHNICAL INFORMATION

Patient ID: Anonymous.
Area: Right leg.
Projection: AP and lateral.
Technical adequacy:

- Inadequate coverage – the entire tibia and fibula have not been included.
- Adequate exposure.
- The patient is not rotated.

● FRACTURE DETAILS

There is a fracture involving the distal tibia.

The fracture is oblique, comminuted and extraarticular, with a longitudinal fracture component in the distal fragment.

There is posterior displacement present along with 90 degrees of external rotation and shortening.

There is no angulation.

There is a fracture involving the proximal fibula.

The fracture is spiral, simple and extraarticular.

There is lateral displacement, medial angulation, 90 degrees of external rotation and shortening.

● JOINTS

There is no subluxation or dislocation.

There are no loose bodies.

There is no effusion or lipohaemarthrosis.

There are no arthritic changes.

● SOFT TISSUES

There is no soft tissue swelling.

There is no surgical emphysema.

● BACKGROUND BONE

The background bone is normal.

● BONE LESIONS

There is no bone lesion present.

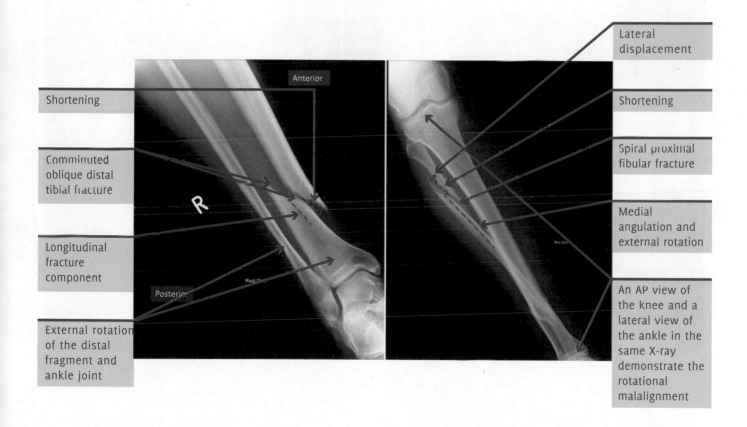

Shortening

Comminuted oblique distal tibial fracture

Longitudinal fracture component

External rotation of the distal fragment and ankle joint

Anterior

R

Posterior

Red Dot

Lateral displacement

Shortening

Spiral proximal fibular fracture

Medial angulation and external rotation

An AP view of the knee and a lateral view of the ankle in the same X-ray demonstrate the rotational malalignment

Red Dot

SUMMARY AND DIFFERENTIAL

Both X-rays demonstrate a right distal third tibial shaft fracture with proximal fibular fracture. There is displacement and angulation, with 90 degrees of external rotation.

INVESTIGATIONS AND MANAGEMENT

Analgesia should be provided.

The fracture should be reduced under sedation. A moulded above-knee back slab should be applied and a CT scan performed to further delineate the fracture and to assess for any distal intraarticular extension.

A referral should be made to orthopaedics for surgical fixation. The patient requires monitoring for compartment syndrome.

A 59-year-old man presents to the ED after he tripped over when getting out of his car. He reports landing directly on his right knee. There is no significant past medical history. On examination, there is tenderness over the joint line of the right knee laterally. There is no ligamentous laxity. Distal pulses are present and motor and sensory function is preserved. The injury is closed.

AP and lateral X-rays of the right knee are requested to assess for a fracture.

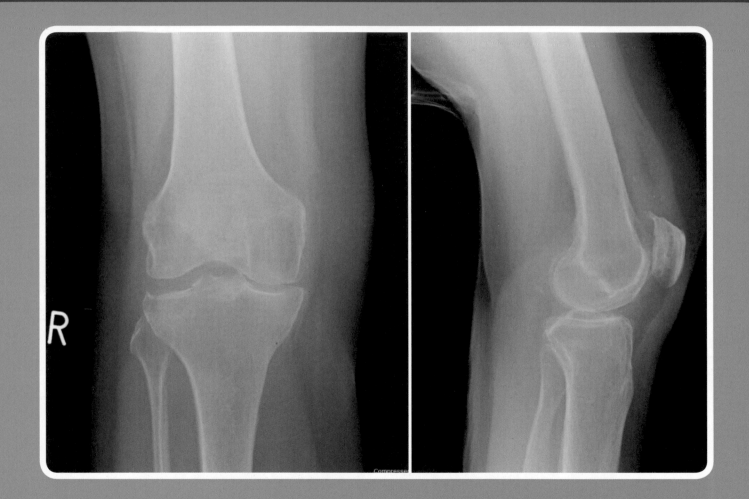

TECHNICAL INFORMATION

Patient ID: Anonymous.
Area: Right knee.
Projection: AP and lateral.
Technical adequacy:

- Adequate coverage.
- Adequate exposure.
- The patient is not rotated.

● FRACTURE DETAILS

There is a fracture involving the lateral plateau of the tibia.

The fracture is longitudinal, simple and intraarticular.

There is approximately 2 mm of depression.

There is no angulation.

There is no rotation.

There is no shortening.

● JOINTS

There is no subluxation or dislocation.

There are no loose bodies.

A knee joint effusion with a fat fluid level is present, which indicates a lipohaemarthrosis.

There are degenerative changes with loss of joint space in the medial and patellofemoral compartments as well as an osteophyte arising from the superior margin of the patella.

● SOFT TISSUES

There is no soft tissue swelling.

There is no surgical emphysema.

● BACKGROUND BONE

The background bone is normal.

● BONE LESIONS

There is no bone lesion present.

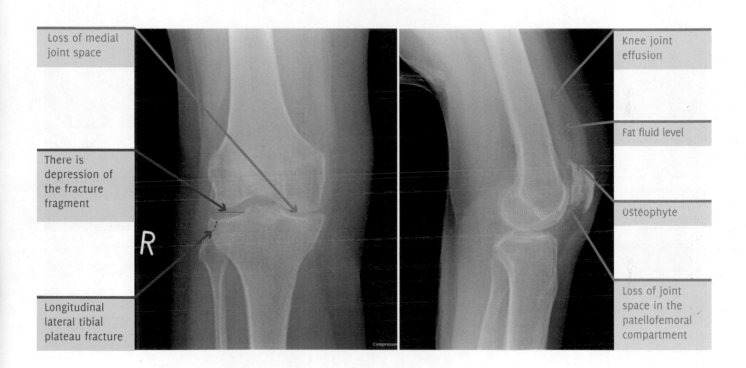

Loss of medial joint space

There is depression of the fracture fragment

R

Longitudinal lateral tibial plateau fracture

Knee joint effusion

Fat fluid level

Osteophyte

Loss of joint space in the patellofemoral compartment

SUMMARY AND DIFFERENTIAL

These X-rays demonstrate a right tibial plateau fracture with lipohaemarthrosis. Involvement of the lateral tibial plateau with depression of the fracture fragment makes this injury a Schatzker type 2 fracture.

INVESTIGATIONS AND MANAGEMENT

Analgesia should be provided.

A cricket pad splint can be applied for comfort. A CT scan should be performed to further assess the fracture and the degree of depression.

A referral should be made to orthopaedics who may consider operative or nonoperative treatment depending on the CT scan findings and discussion with the patient.

A 71-year-old lady has been brought to the ED by her son. She slipped on ice and landed on her left knee. Her knee has since been very painful, and she is struggling to weight bear. There is no significant past medical history. On examination, there is a tender joint line over the left knee with a moderate effusion. The knee is painful through a full range of movement. Distal pulses are present and sensory and motor function is preserved. The injury is closed.

AP and lateral X-rays of the left knee are requested to assess for a fracture.

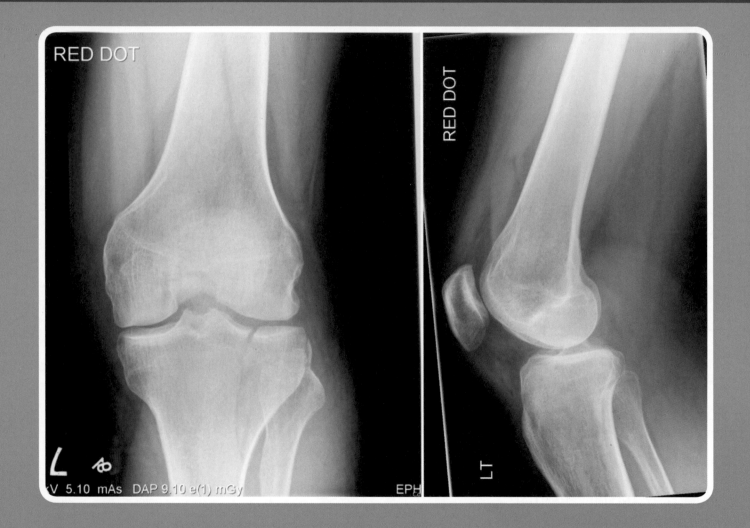

TECHNICAL INFORMATION

Patient ID: Anonymous.
Area: Left knee.
Projection: AP and lateral.
Technical adequacy:

- Adequate coverage.
- Adequate exposure.
- The patient is not rotated.

● FRACTURE DETAILS

There is a fracture involving the lateral plateau of the knee.

The fracture is longitudinal, simple and intraarticular.

There is a gap at the fracture site but no depression.

There is no angulation.

There is no rotation.

There is no shortening.

There is a further avulsion fracture off the margin of the lateral tibial plateau in keeping with an anterolateral ligament avulsion and ACL injury.

● JOINTS

There is no subluxation or dislocation.

There are no loose bodies.

There is a knee joint effusion with a fat fluid level present, which indicates a lipohaemarthrosis.

There are mild degenerative changes with mild joint space loss, particularly in the medial and patellofemoral compartments.

● SOFT TISSUES

There is no soft tissue swelling.

There is no surgical emphysema.

● BACKGROUND BONE

The background bone is normal.

● BONE LESIONS

There is no bone lesion present.

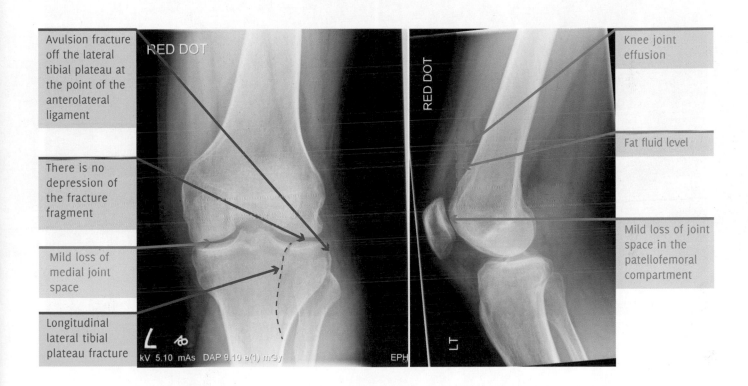

Avulsion fracture off the lateral tibial plateau at the point of the anterolateral ligament

There is no depression of the fracture fragment

Mild loss of medial joint space

Longitudinal lateral tibial plateau fracture

RED DOT

kV 5.10 mAs DAP 9.10 e(1) mGy

RED DOT

Knee joint effusion

Fat fluid level

Mild loss of joint space in the patellofemoral compartment

SUMMARY AND DIFFERENTIAL

Both X-rays demonstrate a right tibial plateau fracture with lipohaemarthrosis. Involvement of the lateral tibial plateau without depression of the fracture fragment makes this injury a Schatzker type 1 fracture. The avulsion fracture off the lateral tibial plateau suggests a concomitant ACL injury.

INVESTIGATIONS AND MANAGEMENT

Analgesia should be provided.

The patient should have the limb placed in a cricket pad splint for comfort. A CT scan should be performed to further delineate the fracture. A referral should be made to orthopaedics who may consider surgical fixation with percutaneous compression screws.

A 77-year-old woman has been referred into hospital by her GP with insidious onset of pain over her distal right leg. She is now unable to weight bear. There is no significant past medical history. Examination of the ankle and knee is normal. There is tenderness over the distal third of the tibia.

AP and lateral X-rays of the right leg are requested to assess for a fracture.

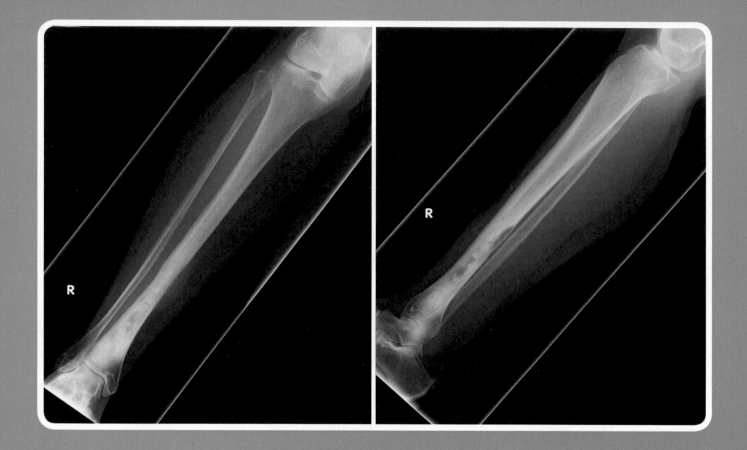

TECHNICAL INFORMATION

Patient ID: Anonymous.
Area: Right leg.
Projection: AP and lateral.
Technical adequacy:

- Adequate coverage.
- Adequate exposure.
- The patient is not rotated.

FRACTURE DETAILS

There is a pathological fracture involving the distal third of the tibia.

The fracture is transverse, simple and extraarticular.

There is no displacement.

There is no angulation.

There is no rotation.

There is no shortening.

JOINTS

There is no subluxation or dislocation.

There are no loose bodies.

There is no effusion or lipohaemarthrosis.

There are mild degenerative changes at the ankle joint, with loss of joint space.

SOFT TISSUES

There is soft tissue swelling/a mass associated with the bone lesion.

There is no surgical emphysema.

BACKGROUND BONE

The background bone is normal.

BONE LESIONS

There is a bone lesion present in the medulla of the distal tibia.

It has a mixed sclerotic and lucent appearance.

There is minimal expansion, best seen on the lateral X-ray.

The zone of transition is wide.

There is cortical thinning posteriorly suggesting bony destruction.

There is no periosteal reaction.

There is a soft tissue mass/component visible.

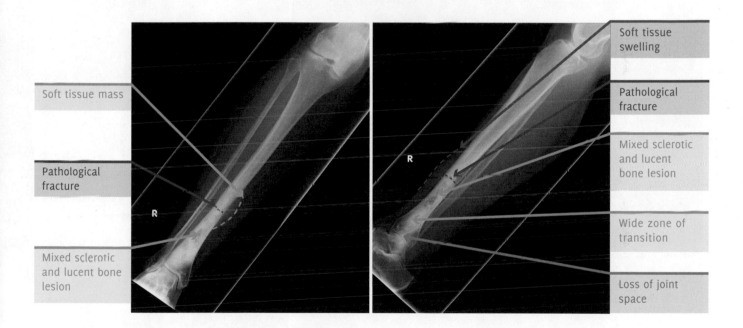

Soft tissue mass

Pathological fracture

Mixed sclerotic and lucent bone lesion

Soft tissue swelling

Pathological fracture

Mixed sclerotic and lucent bone lesion

Wide zone of transition

Loss of joint space

SUMMARY AND DIFFERENTIAL

Both X-rays demonstrate an aggressive appearing bone lesion in the distal tibia. There is an associated undisplaced pathological fracture. The differential diagnosis for the bone lesion includes a primary tumour, such as osteosarcoma, or a metastasis.

INVESTIGATIONS AND MANAGEMENT

Analgesia should be provided.

The lesion should be staged locally with an MRI and distally with a bone scan and a CT scan of the chest, abdomen and pelvis with IV contrast.

Discussion with a specialist bone tumour unit is required.

A 32-year-old man is brought into the regional major trauma centre as a trauma call. He was riding a motorcycle at 40 mph when he struck a van. He fell and trapped his right leg under the motorcycle. There is no significant past medical history. A complete primary survey with CT scan was performed and no major life-threatening injury was identified. On secondary survey, the leg is visibly deformed and swollen. Distal pulses are present, but all movements of the limb are extremely painful and there is altered sensation in the whole foot.

AP and lateral X-rays of the right leg are requested to assess for a fracture.

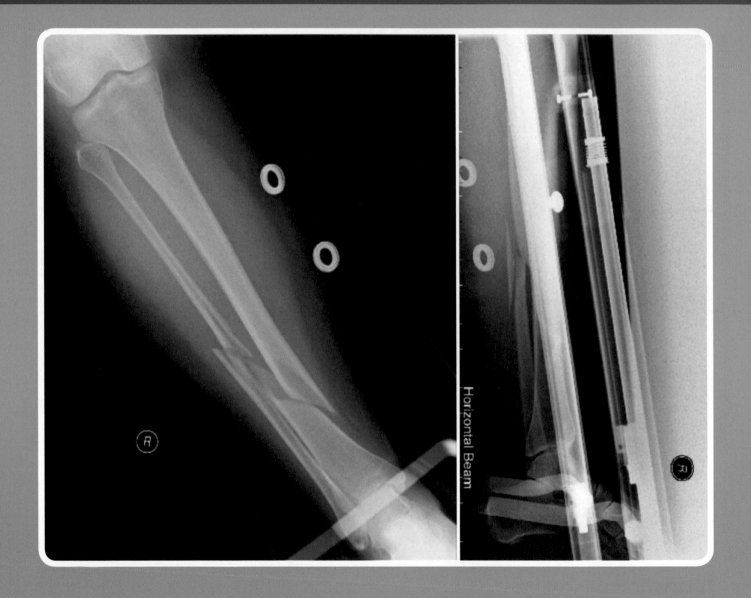

TECHNICAL INFORMATION

Patient ID: Anonymous.
Area: Right leg.
Projection: AP and lateral.
Technical adequacy:

- Inadequate coverage – the tibia and fibula are largely obscured by the metallic splint on the lateral view, and the proximal tibia and fibula are not visible on this view either.
- Adequate exposure.
- The patient is not rotated.

● FRACTURE DETAILS

There is a fracture involving the tibial shaft.

The fracture is spiral, simple and extraarticular.

There is lateral displacement present with some shortening.

There is no angulation.

There is no rotation.

There is a fracture involving the fibular shaft.

The fracture is spiral, comminuted and extraarticular.

There is posterior and lateral displacement present.

There is no angulation.

There is no rotation.

There is some shortening.

● JOINTS

There is no subluxation or dislocation.

There are no loose bodies.

There is no effusion or lipohaemarthrosis.

There are no arthritic changes.

● SOFT TISSUES

There is soft tissue swelling.

There is no surgical emphysema.

● BACKGROUND BONE

The background bone is normal.

● BONE LESIONS

There is no bone lesion present.

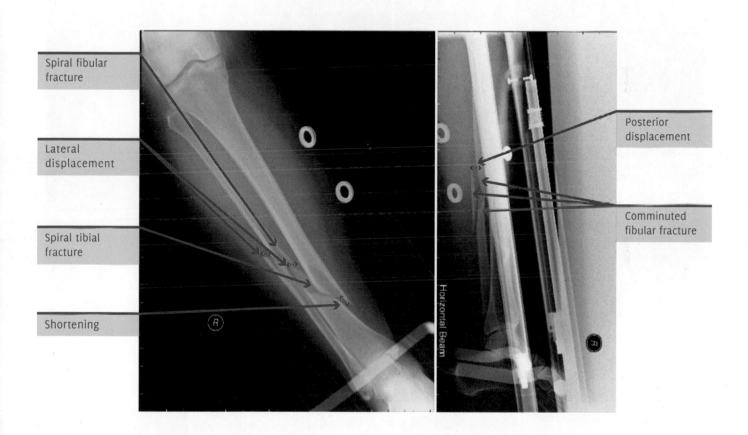

Spiral fibular fracture

Lateral displacement

Spiral tibial fracture

Shortening

Horizontal Beam

Posterior displacement

Comminuted fibular fracture

SUMMARY AND DIFFERENTIAL

Both X-rays demonstrate displaced tibial and fibular spiral shaft fractures. The degree of pain, swelling and altered sensation all fit with a diagnosis of compartment syndrome.

INVESTIGATIONS AND MANAGEMENT

Analgesia should be provided. The patient should be referred to orthopaedics as an emergency. Presuming a diagnosis of compartment syndrome is confirmed, the patient will require fasciotomies and application of external fixation.

A 57-year-old female teacher presents to the ED after she slipped on ice, landing on her left knee. There is no significant past medical history. On examination, there is a boggy swelling over the left knee. The kneecap is tender on palpation and there is a joint effusion. The patient is unable to perform a straight leg raise. Distal pulses are present and sensory and motor function is preserved. The injury is closed.

AP and lateral X-rays of the left knee are requested to assess for a fracture.

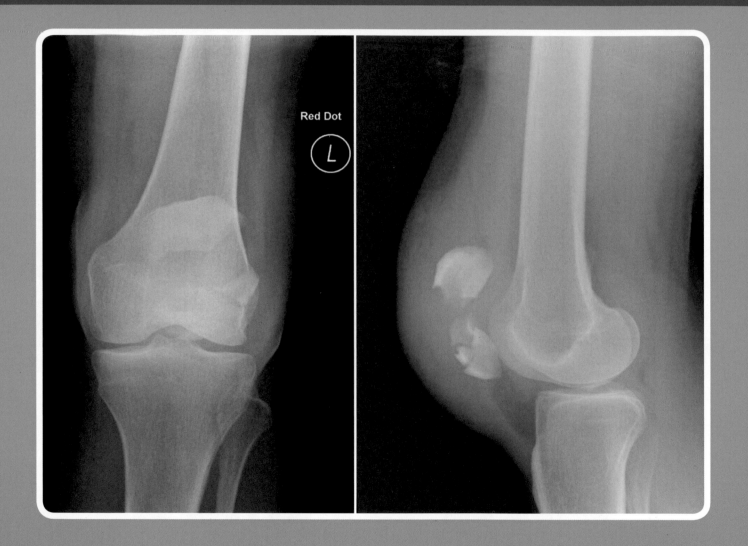

Red Dot

L

TECHNICAL INFORMATION

Patient ID: Anonymous.
Area: Left knee.
Projection: AP mortise and lateral.
Technical adequacy:

- Adequate coverage.
- Adequate exposure.
- The patient is not rotated.

● FRACTURE DETAILS

There is a fracture involving the patella.

The fracture is comminuted and intraarticular.

There is displacement present.

There is no angulation.

There is no rotation.

There is no shortening.

● JOINTS

There is no subluxation or dislocation.

There are no loose bodies.

There is a large lipohaemarthrosis.

There are no arthritic changes.

● SOFT TISSUES

There is marked soft tissue swelling anterior to the knee.

There is no surgical emphysema.

● BACKGROUND BONE

The background bone is normal.

● BONE LESIONS

There is no bone lesion present.

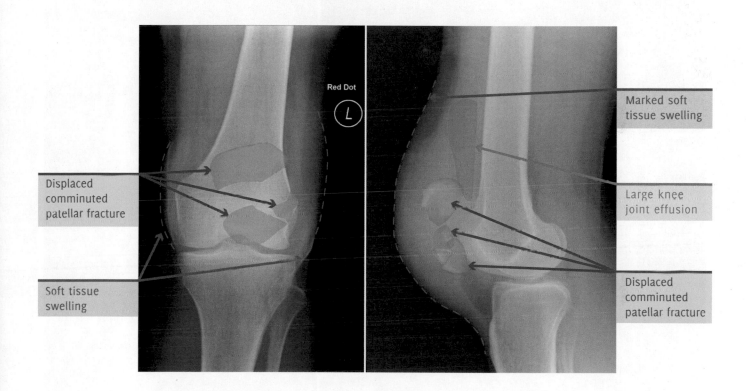

SUMMARY AND DIFFERENTIAL

These X-rays demonstrate a displaced, comminuted patella fracture. This pattern of fracture is referred as a *Stellate (star shaped) fracture*.

INVESTIGATIONS AND MANAGEMENT

Appropriate analgesia should be provided. The leg should be splinted with a cricket pad extension splint.

A referral should be made to an orthopaedic surgeon for surgery. This will consist of ORIF, possibly including the use of tension band wires or cannulated screws.

A 24-year-old woman was tackled whilst playing rugby. She describes sustaining a hyperextension injury to her right knee. She is in severe pain and unable to move her leg. She is brought into the ED by ambulance. There is no significant past medical history. On examination, there is a grossly swollen and deformed knee. The posterior tibial and dorsalis pedis pulses are not palpable. The patient reports altered sensation in the distribution of the common peroneal nerve and is unable to dorsiflex her foot. The injury is closed.

AP and lateral X-rays of the right knee are requested to assess for a fracture or dislocation.

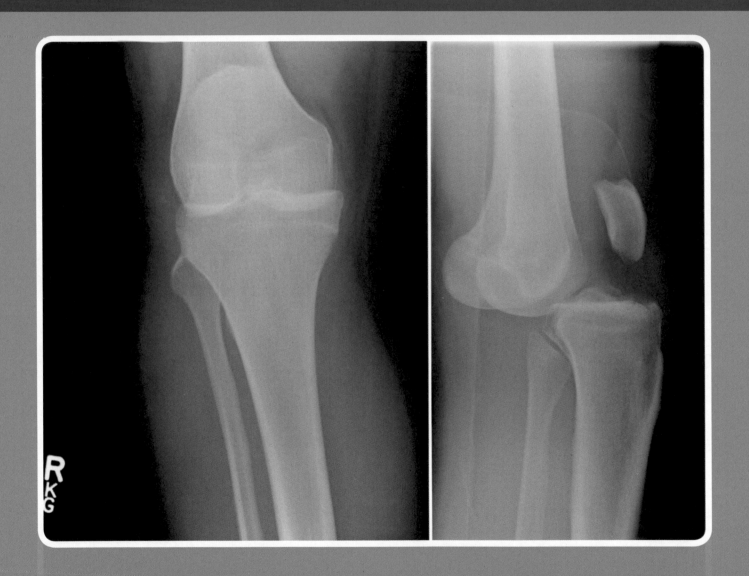

TECHNICAL INFORMATION

Patient ID: Anonymous
Area: Right knee.
Projection: AP and lateral.
Technical adequacy:

- Adequate coverage.
- Adequate exposure.
- The patient is not rotated.

● FRACTURE DETAILS

There is an avulsion fracture of the intercondylar eminence of the tibia.

The fracture is transverse, simple and intraarticular.

There is no displacement.

There is no angulation.

There is no rotation.

There is no shortening.

● JOINTS

There is anterior true knee dislocation of the tibia in relation to the distal femur.

There are no loose bodies.

A knee joint effusion with a fat fluid level can be seen. This is consistent with a lipohaemarthrosis.

There are no arthritic changes.

● SOFT TISSUES

There is no soft tissue swelling.

There is no surgical emphysema.

● BACKGROUND BONE

The background bone is normal.

● BONE LESIONS

There is no bone lesion present.

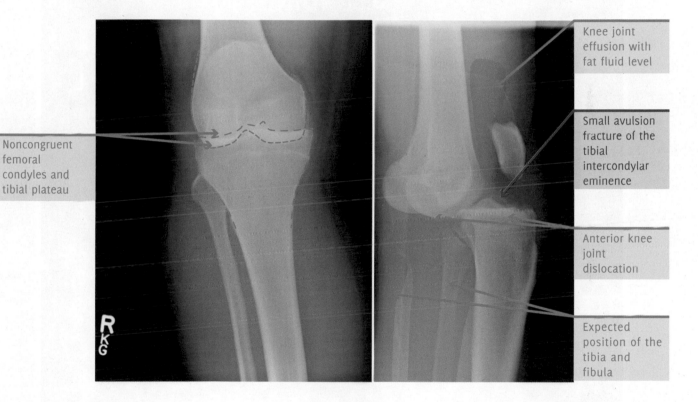

Noncongruent femoral condyles and tibial plateau

Knee joint effusion with fat fluid level

Small avulsion fracture of the tibial intercondylar eminence

Anterior knee joint dislocation

Expected position of the tibia and fibula

SUMMARY AND DIFFERENTIAL

These X-rays demonstrate an anterior true knee dislocation. There is an associated avulsion fracture of the tibial intercondylar eminence at the insertion of the anterior cruciate ligament, with a lipohaemarthrosis.

INVESTIGATIONS AND MANAGEMENT

Appropriate analgesia should be provided.

This is a limb threatening injury. Clear documentation of the pulses and neurological function of the limb is required prior to reduction. Immediate reduction with the assistance of orthopaedics should be performed. Reexamination of the distal pulses and motor and sensory function is required immediately following reduction with clear documentation.

Further management depends on the postreduction examination findings but may include CT angiography and referral to vascular surgery. To understand the full extent of the bony and ligamentous injury, an MRI is required. These are rare, complex injuries, which may require multiple surgeries and months of rehabilitation.

A 40-year-old man presents with a painful swelling over the left knee. He is known to have multiple hereditary exostoses and has had previous surgery on other lesions. He has been to see his GP, who has referred him for a knee X-ray. There is no other significant past medical history. On examination, multiple swellings are visible, and the limb is neutrally aligned.

AP X-rays of both knees while standing are requested to assess for deformity and alignment.

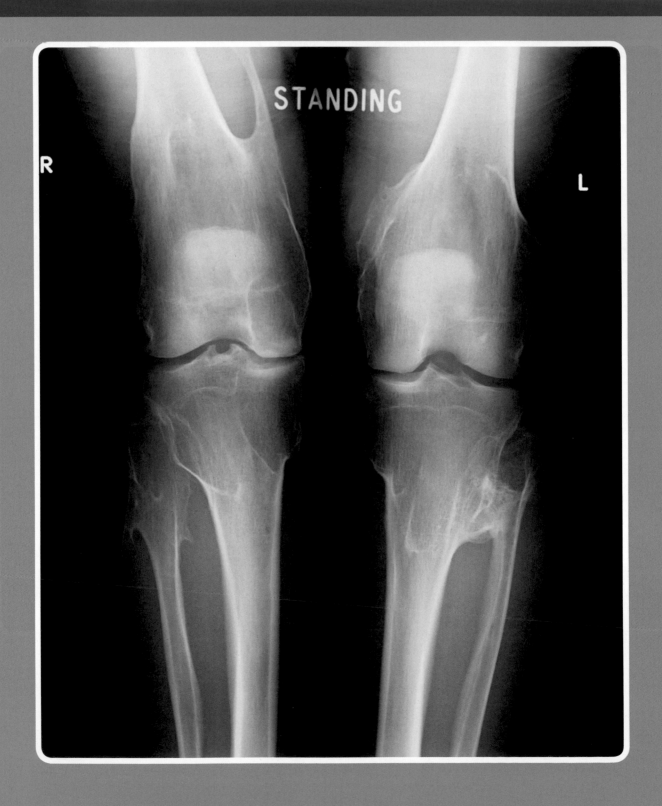

TECHNICAL INFORMATION

Patient ID: Anonymous.
Area: Both knees.
Projection: AP.
Technical adequacy:

- Adequate coverage.
- Adequate exposure.
- The patient is not rotated.

● FRACTURE DETAILS

There is no fracture.

● JOINTS

There is no subluxation or dislocation.

There are no loose bodies.

There is no effusion or lipohaemarthrosis.

There is loss of joint space, subchondral sclerosis and osteophytosis in the medial compartment of the right knee, consistent with degenerative changes.

● SOFT TISSUES

There is no soft tissue swelling.

There is no surgical emphysema.

● BACKGROUND BONE

The background bone demonstrates areas of lucency within the metaphysis of both distal femurs and proximal tibias. These lucent areas are well demarcated with a narrow zone of transition.

● BONE LESIONS

There are multiple bone lesions present in the distal femur and proximal tibia and fibula.

These are expansile and exophytic. Several are pedunculated, while others are sessile.

The zone of transition is narrow and well demarcated.

There is no bony destruction.

There is no periosteal reaction.

There is no soft tissue mass/component visible.

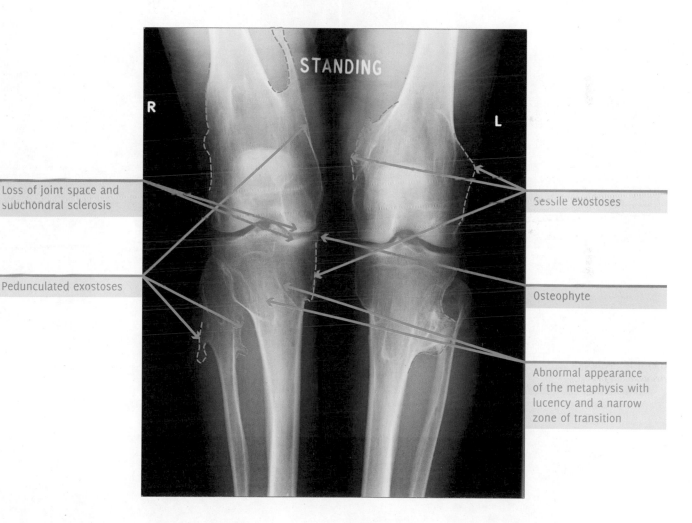

Loss of joint space and subchondral sclerosis

Pedunculated exostoses

STANDING

R

L

Sessile exostoses

Osteophyte

Abnormal appearance of the metaphysis with lucency and a narrow zone of transition

SUMMARY AND DIFFERENTIAL

These X-rays demonstrate multiple well-defined bone lesions without bony destruction or periosteal reaction, in keeping with nonaggressive lesions. The appearances are consistent with multiple exostoses/osteochondromata. The clinical presentation of pain raises clinical suspicion for malignant transformation.

There are also degenerative changes in the right knee joint.

INVESTIGATIONS AND MANAGEMENT

This patient requires an urgent 2-week rule referral to orthopaedics for further imaging in the form of an MRI.

Onward referral to a tertiary bone tumour unit is likely required depending on the results of the scan.

A 22-year-old male student presents to his GP. He was playing football 4 months ago when he jumped for a header and subsequently landed heavily on his feet with high force. For 4 months, he has had ongoing pain over the medial left knee joint line on light exercise with instability and locking. There is no significant past medical history. On examination, there is no effusion or ligamentous laxity. The patient has a full range of movement. On palpation, there is moderate pain localized to the medial joint line.

AP and lateral X-rays of the left knee are requested to assess for a fracture.

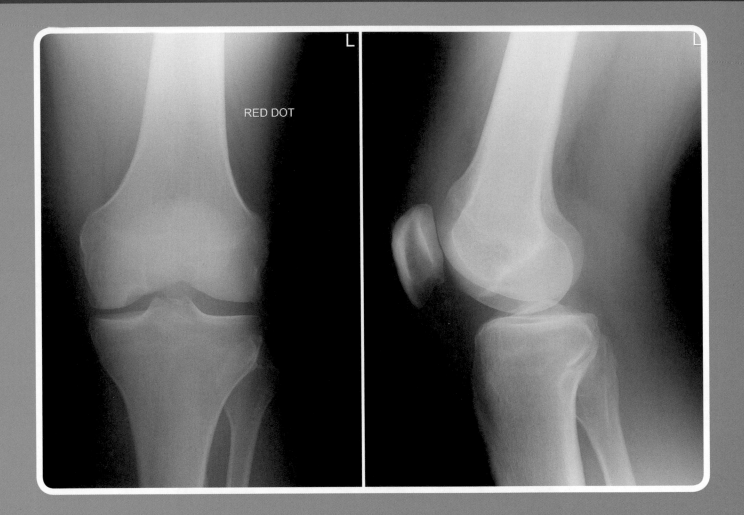

TECHNICAL INFORMATION

Patient ID: Anonymous.
Area: Left knee.
Projection: AP and lateral.
Technical adequacy:

- Adequate coverage.
- Adequate exposure.
- The patient is not rotated.

● FRACTURE DETAILS

There is a defect involving the medial femoral condyle.

It is simple and intraarticular.

The fracture fragment is displaced and rotated, being projected over the lateral aspect of the knee joint.

● JOINTS

There is no subluxation or dislocation.

There is a loose body projected over the lateral aspect of the knee joint.

There is no effusion or lipohaemarthrosis.

There are no arthritic changes.

● SOFT TISSUES

There is no soft tissue swelling.

There is no surgical emphysema.

● BACKGROUND BONE

The background bone is normal.

● BONE LESIONS

There is no bone lesion present.

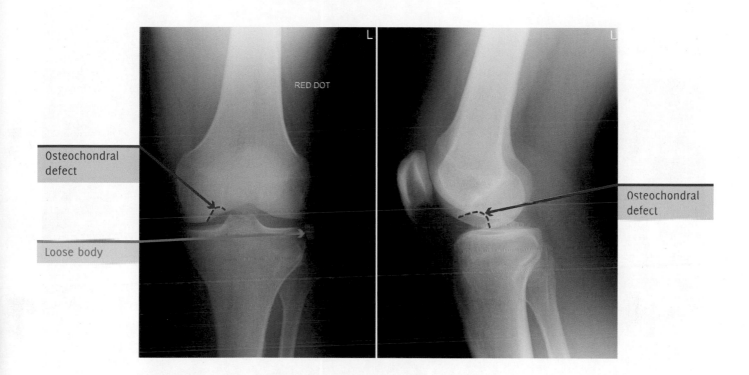

SUMMARY AND DIFFERENTIAL

These X-rays demonstrate an osteochondral defect in the left medial femoral condyle, with an associated loose body.

INVESTIGATIONS AND MANAGEMENT

Appropriate analgesia should be provided.

An MRI should be requested to assess size and position of the osteochondral defect.

A referral should be made to an orthopaedic surgeon who may consider a knee arthroscopy for debridement and microfracture to stimulate cartilage scarring.

A 16-year-old boy twisted his knee whilst playing rugby. He describes feeling his knee give way and subsequently fell to the floor. After this, there was immediate swelling. He has now presented to the orthopaedic trauma clinic. There is no significant past medical history. On examination, there is laxity on the anterior draw test and Lachman test. There is also a moderate effusion. Distal pulses are present and sensory and motor function is preserved.

AP and lateral X-rays of the left knee are requested to assess for a fracture.

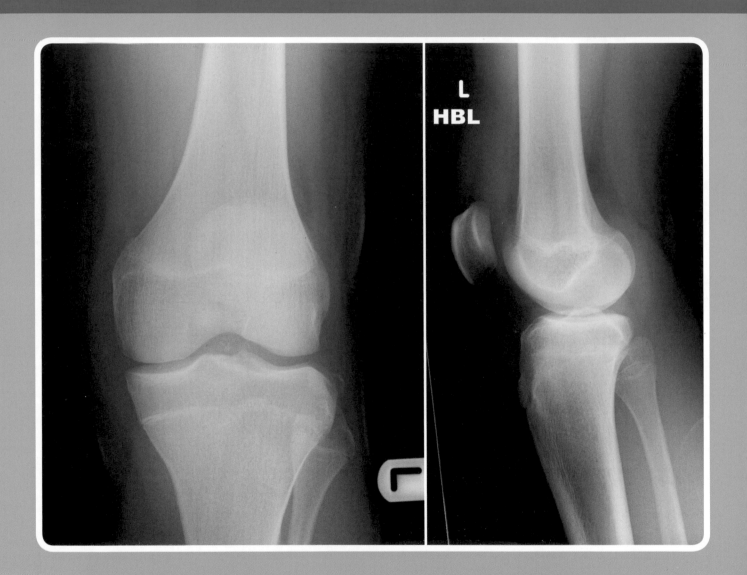

TECHNICAL INFORMATION

Patient ID: Anonymous.
Area: Left knee.
Projection: AP and lateral.
Technical adequacy:

- Adequate coverage.
- Adequate exposure.
- The patient is not rotated.

● FRACTURE DETAILS

There is a fracture involving the lateral aspect of the proximal tibia.

It is longitudinal, simple and intraarticular.

There is minimal displacement present.

There is no angulation.

There is no rotation.

There is no shortening.

● JOINTS

There is no subluxation or dislocation.

There are no loose bodies.

There is a (suprapatellar) knee effusion present.

There are no arthritic changes.

● SOFT TISSUES

There is no soft tissue swelling.

There is no surgical emphysema.

● BACKGROUND BONE

The background bone is normal.

● BONE LESIONS

There is no bone lesion present.

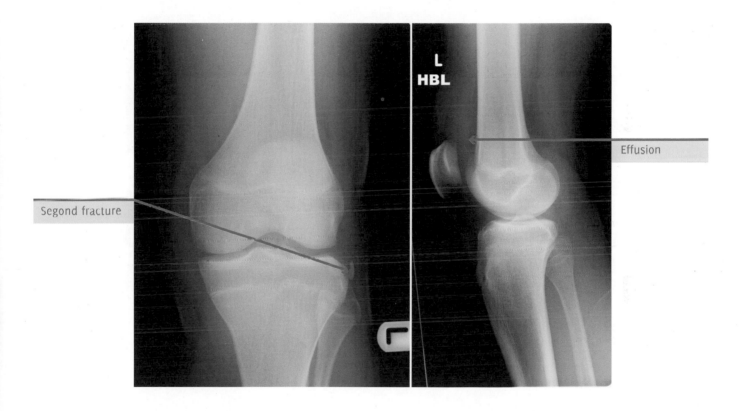

SUMMARY AND DIFFERENTIAL

These X-rays demonstrate a minimally displaced fracture of the lateral tibial plateau. The findings are consistent with a Segond fracture, which is pathognomic for an anterior cruciate ligament rupture.

INVESTIGATIONS AND MANAGEMENT

RICE should be encouraged initially followed by range of movement exercises.

An MRI scan should be requested to assess the knee ligaments.

A referral should be made to an orthopaedic surgeon who may consider ACL reconstruction.

A 75-year-old former dock worker presents to his GP with several weeks' history of a sore left ankle. He thinks he may have fallen and twisted it but is uncertain. He is struggling to weight bear. He has recently been diagnosed with lung cancer. On examination, the patient walks with an antalgic gait on the left and has tenderness over the left lateral malleolus. The foot is neurovascularly intact. The injury is closed.

AP and lateral X-rays of the left ankle are requested to assess for a fracture.

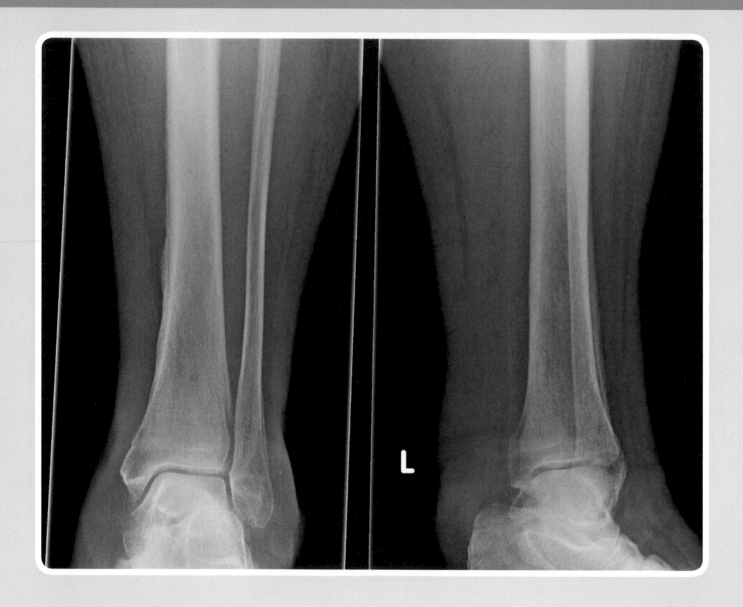

TECHNICAL INFORMATION

Patient ID: Anonymous.
Area: Left ankle.
Projection: AP and lateral.
Technical adequacy:

- Adequate coverage.
- Adequate exposure.
- The patient is rotated on the lateral view.

● FRACTURE DETAILS

There is no fracture.

● JOINTS

There is no subluxation or dislocation.

There are no loose bodies.

There is no effusion or lipohaemarthrosis.

There are no arthritic changes.

● SOFT TISSUES

There is no soft tissue swelling.

There is no surgical emphysema.

● BACKGROUND BONE

The background bone is normal, except for the periosteum.

● BONE LESIONS

There is thick periosteal reaction involving the lateral and anterior aspects of the left distal tibia and fibula respectively (diaphysis and metaphysis).

There is no associated bone lesion visible.

There is no bony destruction.

There is no soft tissue mass/component visible.

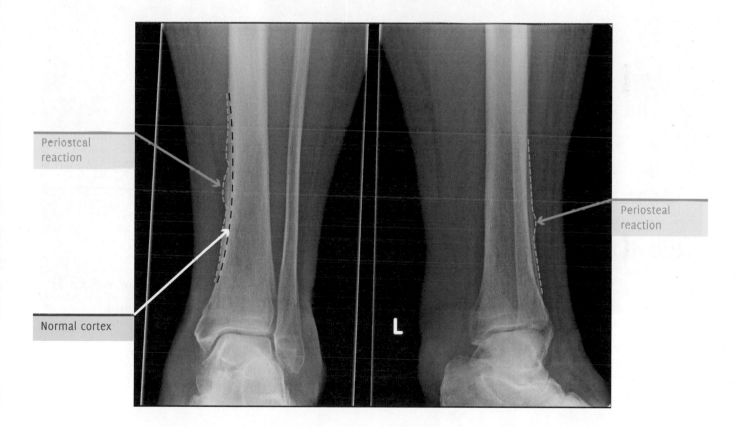

Periosteal reaction

Normal cortex

Periosteal reaction

L

SUMMARY AND DIFFERENTIAL

Both X-rays demonstrate a thick periosteal reaction affecting the distal tibia and fibula. The findings most likely represent a hypertrophic osteoarthropathy. It is likely to be related to a lung carcinoma and would account for the patient's symptoms. The differential diagnosis for hypertrophic osteoarthropathy includes other pulmonary and pleural conditions, such as lung abscess, bronchiectasis, mesothelioma, and gastrointestinal conditions, such as inflammatory bowel disease. There is no fracture or discrete bone lesion visible.

INVESTIGATIONS AND MANAGEMENT

Advice regarding analgesia should be provided.

There is no specific treatment for hypertrophic osteoarthropathy other than analgesia.

A 72-year-old man has been brought to the ED after he fell down a grassy bank whilst walking his dog. He is complaining of pain and an inability to weight bear on his right ankle. There is a past medical history of heart failure. On examination, the patient is tender over the distal tibia and fibula. The distal tibia is palpably mobile. Distal pulses are present and sensory and motor function is preserved. The injury is closed.

AP and lateral X-rays of the right ankle are requested to assess for a fracture.

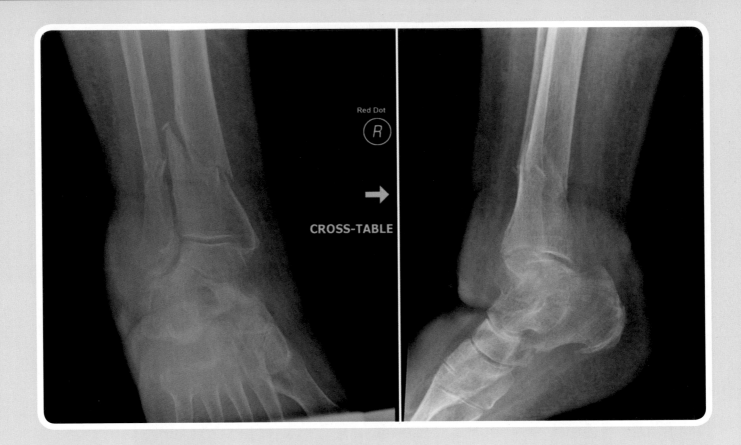

Red Dot

(R)

→

CROSS-TABLE

TECHNICAL INFORMATION

Patient ID: Anonymous.
Area: Right ankle.
Projection: AP and lateral.
Technical adequacy:

- Adequate coverage.
- Adequate exposure.
- The patient is not rotated.

● FRACTURE DETAILS

There is a fracture involving the distal tibia.

The fracture is oblique, comminuted and extraarticular.

There is lateral displacement, minor posterior angulation and minimal shortening.

There is no rotation.

There is a fracture involving the distal fibula.

The fracture is transverse, comminuted and extraarticular.

There is no displacement.

Minor lateral angulation is present.

There is no rotation.

There is no shortening.

● JOINTS

There is no subluxation or dislocation.

There are no loose bodies.

There is no effusion or lipohaemarthrosis.

There is osteoarthritis of the ankle.

● SOFT TISSUES

There is generalized soft tissue swelling, probably related to heart failure.

There is no surgical emphysema.

● BACKGROUND BONE

The background bone is osteopenic.

● BONE LESIONS

There is no bone lesion present.

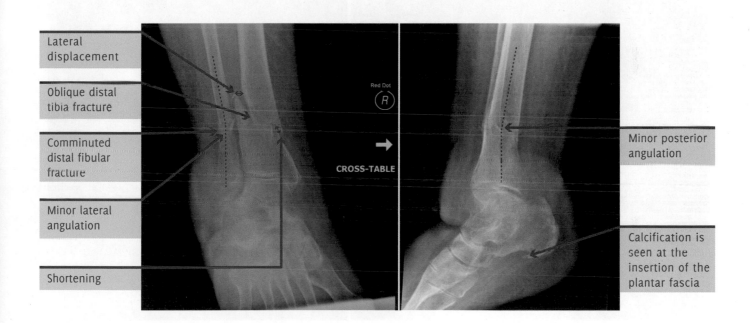

Lateral displacement

Oblique distal tibia fracture

Comminuted distal fibular fracture

Minor lateral angulation

Shortening

Red Dot
(R)
→ CROSS-TABLE

Minor posterior angulation

Calcification is seen at the insertion of the plantar fascia

SUMMARY AND DIFFERENTIAL

Both X-rays demonstrate minimally displaced right distal tibia and fibula fractures.

INVESTIGATIONS AND MANAGEMENT

Advice regarding analgesia should be provided.

The patient should have a back slab applied in the ED. A CT scan should be performed to assess for intraarticular extension and to further delineate the fracture. A referral should be made to orthopaedics for surgical fixation.

A 39-year-old female presents to the ED having sustained an inversion injury to her left ankle. There is no significant past medical history. On examination, there is moderate swelling and tenderness over the lateral malleolus. There is no medial tenderness. Movement at the ankle is restricted in all directions. She cannot weight bear. Distal pulses are present and sensory and motor function is preserved. The injury is closed.

AP mortise and lateral X-rays of the left ankle are requested to assess for a fracture.

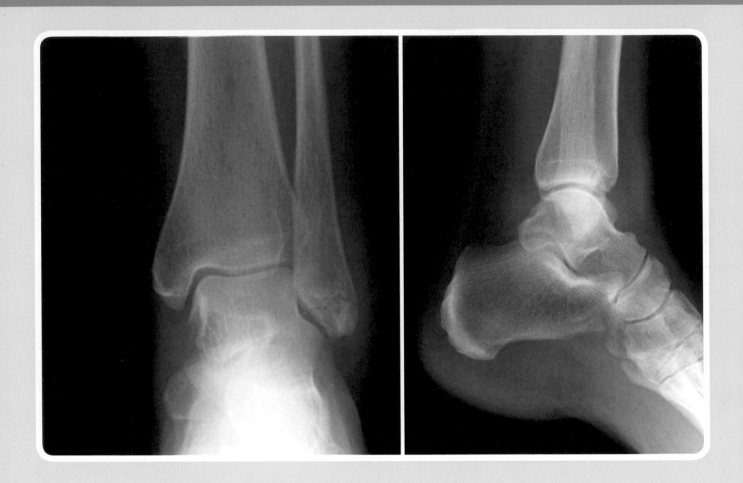

TECHNICAL INFORMATION

Patient ID: Anonymous.
Area: Left ankle.
Projection: AP mortise and lateral.
Technical adequacy:

- Adequate coverage.
- Adequate exposure.
- The patient is not rotated.

● FRACTURE DETAILS

There is an ankle fracture affecting the distal third of the fibula.

The fracture is transverse, simple and intraarticular.

There is no displacement.

There is no angulation.

There is no rotation.

There is no shortening.

● JOINTS

There is no widening of the tibiofibular or medial clear spaces (both <5 mm).

There is no subluxation or dislocation.

There are no loose bodies.

There is no effusion or lipohaemarthrosis.

There are no arthritic changes.

The mortise is intact, that is, plafond normal, talus is undisplaced, no widening of the syndesmosis.

● SOFT TISSUES

There is soft tissue swelling over the anterior and lateral ankle joint.

There is no surgical emphysema.

● BACKGROUND BONE

The background bone is normal.

● BONE LESIONS

There is no bone lesion present.

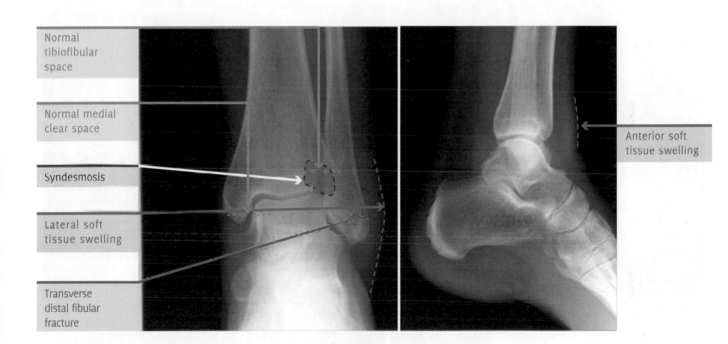

Normal tibiofibular space

Normal medial clear space

Syndesmosis

Lateral soft tissue swelling

Transverse distal fibular fracture

Anterior soft tissue swelling

SUMMARY AND DIFFERENTIAL

These X-rays demonstrate an isolated, undisplaced fracture of the distal fibula. The fracture is below the level of the syndesmosis and is therefore consistent with a Weber A ankle fracture.

INVESTIGATIONS AND MANAGEMENT

Appropriate analgesia should be provided.

Either a walking boot or below-knee back slab should be applied.

Crutches should be supplied, and the patient should be allowed to weight bear on the ankle as pain allows. The patient should be given RICE advice.

A referral should be made to the local fracture clinic for routine follow-up.

A 43-year-old teacher presents to the Minor Injuries Unit having slipped on wet leaves at school. She thinks she has twisted her right ankle. There is no significant past medical history. On examination, there is significant swelling and bruising over both the medial and lateral malleoli, with inability to weight bear. Distal pulses are present and sensory and motor function is preserved. The injury is closed.

AP mortise and lateral X-rays of the right ankle are requested to assess for a fracture.

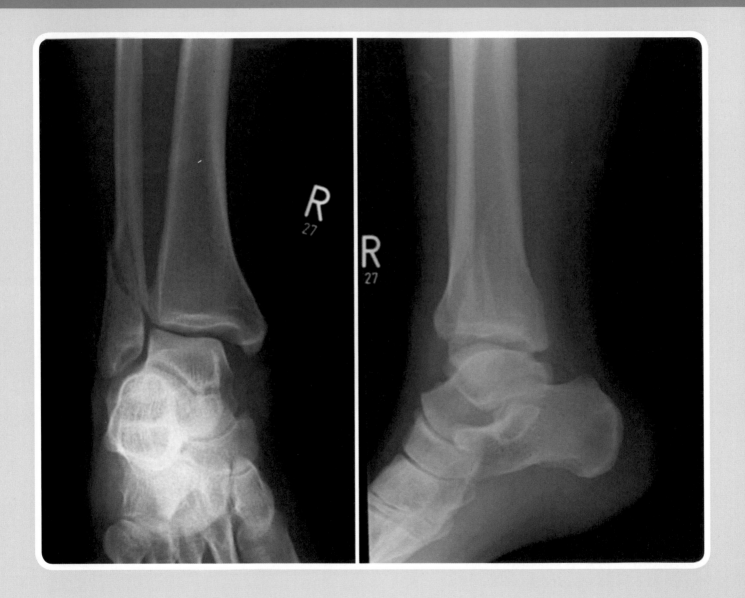

TECHNICAL INFORMATION

Patient ID: Anonymous.
Area: Right ankle.
Projection: AP mortise and lateral.
Technical adequacy:

- Adequate coverage.
- Adequate exposure.
- The patient is not rotated.

● FRACTURE DETAILS

There is an ankle fracture involving the distal third of the fibula.

The fracture is spiral, simple and intraarticular.

There is lateral and posterior displacement of the distal fracture fragment.

There is no angulation.

There is external rotation.

There is shortening.

● JOINTS

There is a 5-mm lateral talar shift, resulting in widened medial clear space. The tibiofibular clear space is difficult to assess.

There is lateral subluxation of the talus relative to the tibia.

There are no loose bodies.

There is no effusion or lipohaemarthrosis.

There are no arthritic changes.

● SOFT TISSUES

There is medial, lateral and anterior soft tissue swelling.

There is no surgical emphysema.

● BACKGROUND BONE

The background bone is normal.

● BONE LESIONS

There is no bone lesion present.

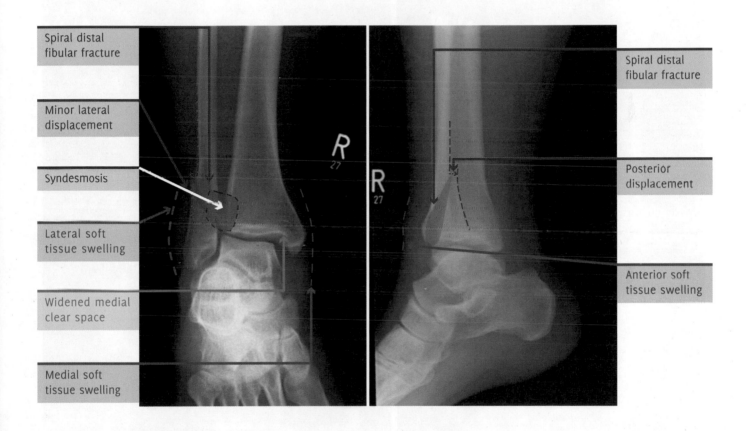

Spiral distal fibular fracture	
Minor lateral displacement	
Syndesmosis	
Lateral soft tissue swelling	
Widened medial clear space	
Medial soft tissue swelling	
	Spiral distal fibular fracture
	Posterior displacement
	Anterior soft tissue swelling

SUMMARY AND DIFFERENTIAL

These X-rays demonstrate a spiral fracture of the distal fibula with lateral and posterior displacement. The fracture is at the level of the syndesmosis and is therefore consistent with a Weber B ankle fracture.

INVESTIGATIONS AND MANAGEMENT

Appropriate analgesia should be provided.

The patient should undergo reduction under sedation in the ED.

A moulded back slab should be applied and an X-ray taken to check positioning.

This fracture is unstable as demonstrated by the talar shift. This is best treated surgically unless there is a medical contraindication.

A referral should be made to the orthopaedic team for further management. This may include ORIF with fibula lag screw, neutralization plate and intraoperative syndesmosis assessment.

Weight bearing after surgery will be the surgeon's choice but where bone quality and fixation is good then early weight bearing in a walking boot is achievable.

A 28-year-old woman presents to the ED having slipped down three steps while at a party under the influence of alcohol. Following the fall, she has been unable to stand as she complains of pain in her left ankle. There is no significant past medical history. On examination, there is marked pain, swelling and bruising over both the medial and lateral malleoli with an obvious clinical deformity and medial skin tenting. This is suggestive of a fracture and dislocation. However, the injury is closed. The foot has a dusky appearance and distal pulses are only identified on doppler. Distal sensation is intact. Motor assessment is not possible secondary to pain.

AP mortise and lateral X-rays of the left ankle are requested to assess for a fracture.

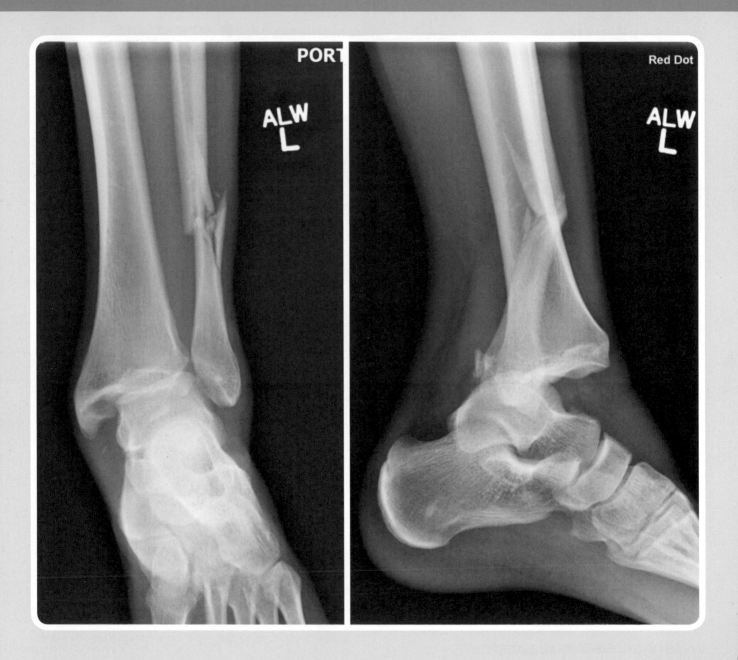

TECHNICAL INFORMATION

Patient ID: Anonymous.
Area: Left ankle.
Projection: AP mortise and lateral.
Technical adequacy:

- Adequate coverage.
- Adequate exposure.
- The patient is not rotated.

● FRACTURE DETAILS

There is a fracture of the distal third of the fibula.

The fracture is oblique, comminuted and intraarticular.

There is lateral displacement.

There is posterior angulation.

There is rotation.

There is ~3 mm of fibula shortening.

There is possibly a displaced fracture of the posterior malleolus, although it is difficult to assess.

● JOINTS

There is posterior dislocation of the tibiotalar (ankle) joint.

There is widening of the medial clear space (talar shift) and the tibiofibular clear space suggesting disruption of the syndesmosis.

There are no loose bodies.

There is no effusion or lipohaemarthrosis.

There are no arthritic changes.

● SOFT TISSUES

There is medial skin tenting.

There is no surgical emphysema.

● BACKGROUND BONE

The background bone is normal.

● BONE LESIONS

There is no bone lesion present.

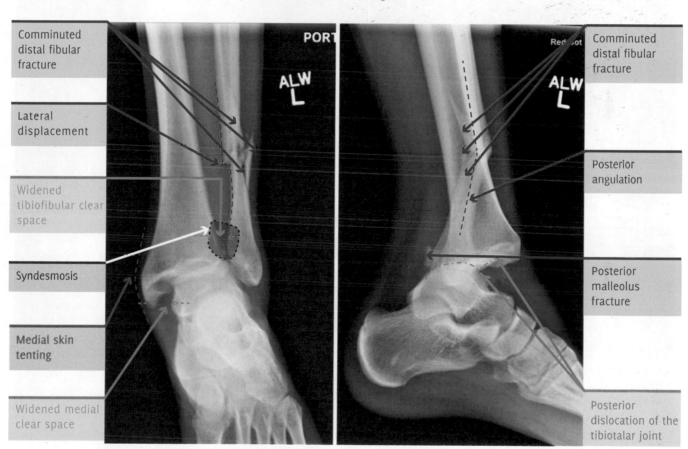

Left image labels: Comminuted distal fibular fracture; Lateral displacement; Widened tibiofibular clear space; Syndesmosis; Medial skin tenting; Widened medial clear space

Right image labels: Comminuted distal fibular fracture; Posterior angulation; Posterior malleolus fracture; Posterior dislocation of the tibiotalar joint

SUMMARY AND DIFFERENTIAL

Both X-rays demonstrate a displaced and comminuted ankle fracture involving the distal fibula with posterior angulation and fibula shortening. There is dislocation of the tibiotalar (ankle) joint. The fracture is above the level of the syndesmosis and is therefore consistent with a Weber C ankle fracture. There is an associated fracture of the posterior malleolus.

INVESTIGATIONS AND MANAGEMENT

Appropriate analgesia should be provided.

The patient should undergo reduction under sedation in the ED as an emergency, as this is a limb-threatening injury. It may be appropriate to refer to orthopaedics to assist with the reduction.

A moulded back slab should be applied.

Following reduction, distal pulses, sensory and motor function should be reassessed and documented.

The limb should be elevated, and a CT scan performed to check positioning and to fully understand this complex injury for surgical planning. A referral to the on-call orthopaedic team is required. Surgical management may include ORIF with plate and screw plus syndesmosis fixation.

A 68-year-old woman attends the ED after slipping at the supermarket. She thinks she has twisted her left ankle. She has a past history of hypertension. On examination, there is swelling and tenderness over the medial and lateral malleoli. She is unable to move her foot without significant pain and cannot weight bear. The skin quality appears poor but distal pulses are present and distal sensory and motor function is intact. The injury is closed.

AP mortise and lateral X-rays of the left ankle are requested to assess for a fracture.

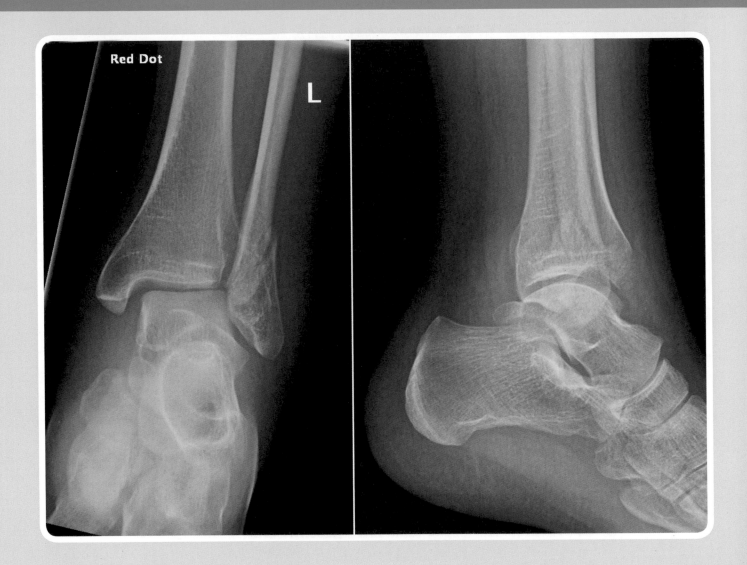

Red Dot

L

TECHNICAL INFORMATION

Patient ID: Anonymous.
Area: Left ankle.
Projection: AP mortise and lateral.
Technical adequacy:

- Adequate coverage.
- Adequate exposure.
- The patient is not rotated.

● FRACTURE DETAILS

There is a fracture involving the distal third of the fibula.

The fracture is oblique, simple and extraarticular.

There is minor lateral and posterior displacement.

There is no angulation.

There is external rotation of the distal fragment.

There is no shortening.

There also appears to be a fracture of the anterior aspect of the distal tibia.

The fracture is simple and intraarticular.

There is superior displacement and angulation.

There is no rotation.

● JOINTS

There is widening of the medial clear space (talar shift). The tibiofibular clear space is normal.

There are no loose bodies.

There is no effusion or lipohaemarthrosis.

There are no arthritic changes.

● SOFT TISSUES

There is medial skin tenting.

There is no surgical emphysema.

● BACKGROUND BONE

The background bone is normal.

● BONE LESIONS

There is no bone lesion present.

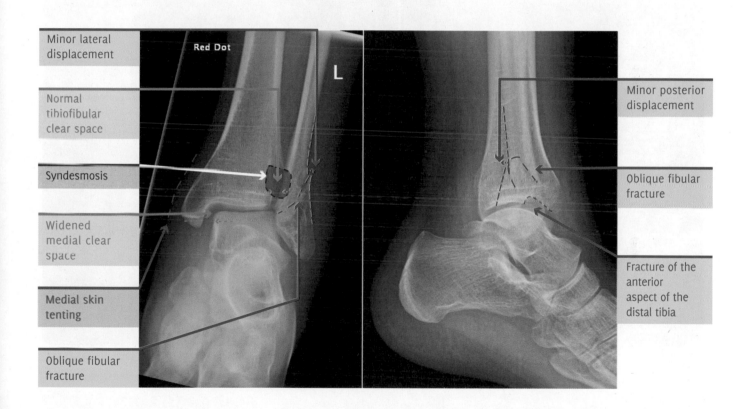

Minor lateral displacement	Red Dot
Normal tibiofibular clear space	Minor posterior displacement
Syndesmosis	Oblique fibular fracture
Widened medial clear space	
Medial skin tenting	Fracture of the anterior aspect of the distal tibia
Oblique fibular fracture	

SUMMARY AND DIFFERENTIAL

Both X-rays demonstrate a displaced fracture of the distal fibula with talar shift. There may also be a distal tibial fracture anteriorly. The fibula fracture is at the level of the syndesmosis and is therefore consistent with a Weber B ankle fracture.

INVESTIGATIONS AND MANAGEMENT

Appropriate analgesia should be provided.

The ankle should be reduced under sedation in the ED.

A moulded back slab should be applied and a CT scan performed to check positioning and further assess the distal tibia.

This is an unstable fracture with talar shift and is therefore best treated surgically. A referral should be made to the orthopaedic team.

Surgical options include ORIF with fibula plate fixation and lag screw. Intraoperative stress tests should be conducted to determine if a syndesmosis screw is required.

A 19-year-old male presents to the ED after everting his right ankle when landing during a rugby lineout. He is unable to weight bear. There is no significant past medical history. On examination, there is minor swelling around the medial aspect of the right ankle and limited movement. There is also pain at the right knee. Distal pulses are present and sensory and motor function is preserved. The injury is closed.

AP and lateral X-rays of the right ankle and fibula are requested to assess for a fracture.

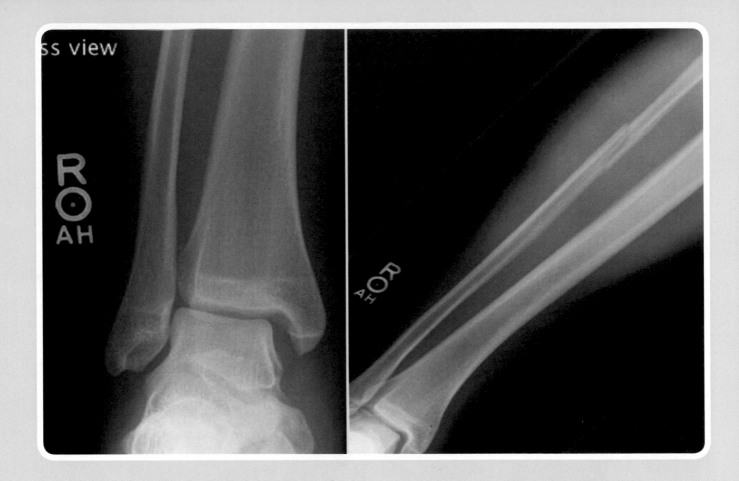

TECHNICAL INFORMATION

Patient ID: Anonymous.
Area: Right ankle and proximal fibula.
Projection: AP mortise and AP mid-fibula.
Technical adequacy:

- The medial soft tissues of the ankle have not been fully included on the AP mortise view. The proximal fibula has not been included and lateral views are not presented.
- Adequate exposure.
- The patient is not rotated.

● FRACTURE DETAILS

There is a fracture involving the proximal third of the fibula.

The fracture is spiral, simple and extraarticular.

There is minimal lateral displacement. Anterior/posterior displacement cannot be assessed on these views.

There is no angulation.

There is no rotation.

There is no shortening.

● JOINTS

There is widening of the medial clear space (talar shift) and tibiofibular clear space.

There are no loose bodies.

There is no effusion or lipohaemarthrosis.

There are no arthritic changes.

● SOFT TISSUES

There is no soft tissue swelling.

There is no surgical emphysema.

● BACKGROUND BONE

The background bone is normal.

● BONE LESIONS

There is no bone lesion present.

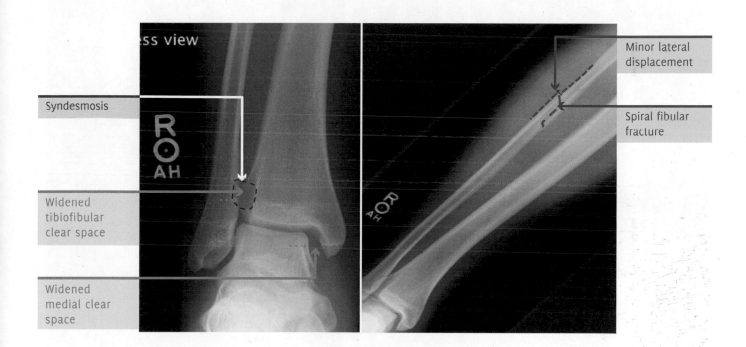

Syndesmosis

Widened tibiofibular clear space

Widened medial clear space

Minor lateral displacement

Spiral fibular fracture

SUMMARY AND DIFFERENTIAL

These X-rays demonstrate an ankle injury with a minimally displaced proximal fibular fracture. Widening of the medial and tibiofibular clear spaces indicate deltoid ligament and tibiofibular syndesmosis disruption. The injury pattern is consistent with a Maisonneuve fracture.

INVESTIGATIONS AND MANAGEMENT

Appropriate analgesia should be provided.

Reduction should be performed under sedation in the ED.

A moulded back slab should be applied and an X-ray taken to check positioning.

A referral should be made to the orthopaedic team for surgical management. This may include CRIF with syndesmosis screw fixation.

A 68-year-old male presents to the ED by ambulance having fallen 4 feet from a loft hatch onto his left ankle. He has a past medical history of gastrooesophageal reflux disease and hypertension. On examination, there is an obvious deformity of the left ankle with medial skin tenting and bruising and he is unable to move it. The foot is dusky in appearance with pulses identified on doppler. The patient reports altered sensation in the foot, and it is not possible to assess motor function secondary to pain. The injury is closed.

AP mortise and lateral X-rays of the left ankle are requested to assess for fracture.

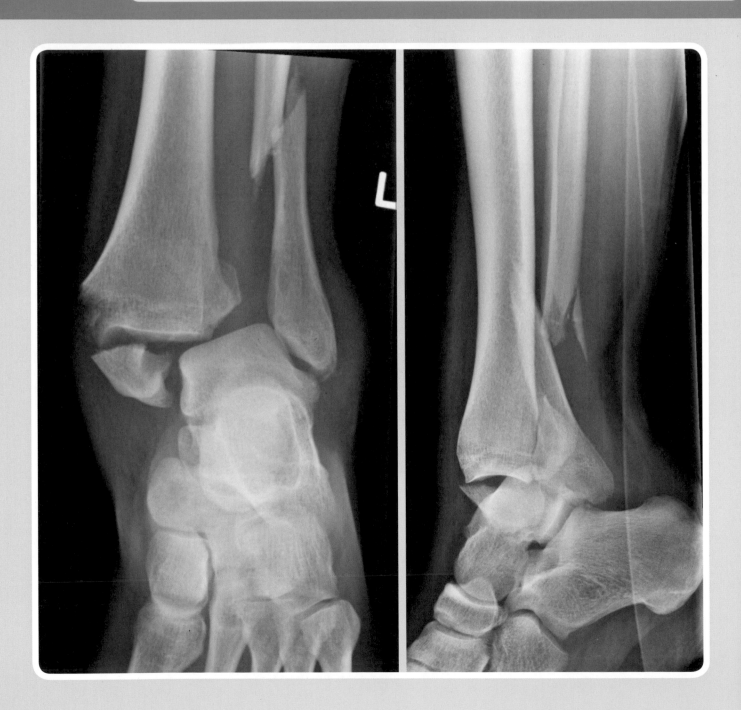

TECHNICAL INFORMATION

Patient ID: Anonymous.
Area: Left ankle.
Projection: AP mortise and lateral.
Technical adequacy:

- Adequate coverage.
- Adequate exposure.
- The patient is not rotated.

● FRACTURE DETAILS

There is a fracture to the distal third of the fibula.

The fracture is oblique, comminuted and extraarticular.

There is marked anterior and lateral displacement.

There is posterior angulation of the fibula.

There is no rotation.

There is shortening of the fibula.

There is a fracture to the medial malleolus.

The fracture is longitudinal, simple and intraarticular.

There is lateral and inferior displacement.

There is no angulation.

The distal fragment is rotated 90 degrees.

There is no shortening.

There is a fracture to the posterior malleolus.

The fracture is longitudinal, simple and intraarticular.

There is displacement.

There is no angulation.

There is no rotation.

There is shortening.

● JOINTS

There is posterior and lateral dislocation of the tibiotalar joint with marked widening of the medial and tibiofibular clear spaces.

There are no loose bodies.

There is no effusion or lipohaemarthrosis.

There are no arthritic changes.

● SOFT TISSUES

There is anterior and medial skin tenting.

There is no surgical emphysema.

● BACKGROUND BONE

The background bone is normal.

● BONE LESIONS

There is no bone lesion present.

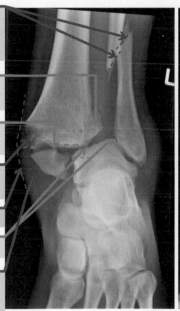
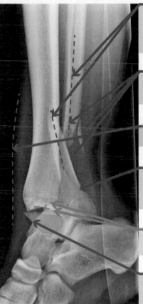

Oblique distal fibular fracture with shortening and lateral displacement

Markedly widened tibiofibular clear space

Markedly widened medial clear space

Longitudinal medial malleolus fracture

Medial skin tenting

Lateral tibiotalar dislocation

Displaced and rotated medial malleolus fracture fragment

Anterior displacement, posterior angulation and shortening

Comminuted distal fibular fracture

Anterior skin tenting

Undisplaced posterior malleolus fracture fragment

Posterior tibiotalar dislocation

Medial malleolus fracture fragment

SUMMARY AND DIFFERENTIAL

Both X-rays demonstrate a trimalleolar ankle fracture with dislocation of the tibiotalar joint.

INVESTIGATIONS AND MANAGEMENT

Appropriate analgesia should be provided.

A fall from height such as this should raise alarm for other injuries and the patient should be initially managed as a trauma call with an ATLS protocol.

Once life-threatening injuries have been excluded, the patient should undergo reduction under sedation in the ED as an emergency as this is a limb-threatening injury. It may be appropriate to refer to orthopaedics to assist with the reduction.

A moulded back slab should be applied.

Following reduction, distal pulses, sensory and motor function should be reassessed and documented.

The limb should be elevated, and a CT scan performed to check positioning and to fully understand this complex injury for surgical planning. A referral to the on-call orthopaedic team is required.

Surgical management may include ORIF of the fibula with plate and screw plus syndesmosis fixation, screw fixation of the medial malleolus and possible fixation of the posterior malleolus.

A 21-year-old female presents to the Minor Injuries Unit after twisting her left ankle while playing netball. She is unable to weight bear. She has a past medical history of asthma. On examination, there is swelling over the medial malleolus and restricted movement. There is no proximal fibula pain. Distal pulses are present and motor and sensory function is preserved. The injury is closed.

AP mortise and lateral X-rays of the left ankle are requested to assess for a fracture.

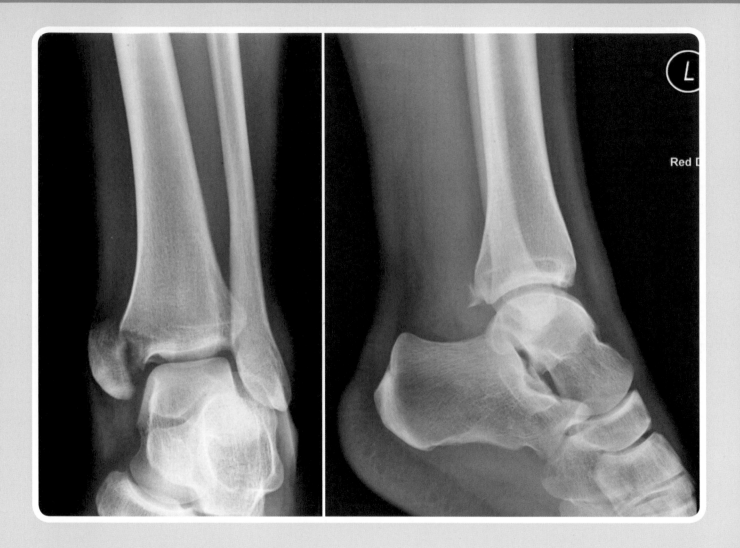

TECHNICAL INFORMATION

Patient ID: Anonymous.
Area: Left ankle.
Projection: AP mortise and lateral.
Technical adequacy:

- Adequate coverage.
- Adequate exposure.
- The patient is not rotated.

● FRACTURE DETAILS

There is a fracture to the medial malleolus.

The fracture is longitudinal, simple and intraarticular.

There is medial displacement.

There is angulation.

There is rotation.

There is shortening.

There is an associated fracture of the posterior malleolus.

The fracture appears longitudinal, simple and intraarticular although the exact nature of the posterior malleolar fracture cannot be identified.

There is minor posterior displacement.

There is no angulation.

There is no rotation.

There is no shortening.

● JOINTS

There is no subluxation or dislocation.

There are no loose bodies.

There is no effusion or lipohaemarthrosis.

There are no arthritic changes.

● SOFT TISSUES

There is medial skin tenting and soft tissue swelling.

There is no surgical emphysema.

● BACKGROUND BONE

The background bone is normal.

● BONE LESIONS

There is no bone lesion present.

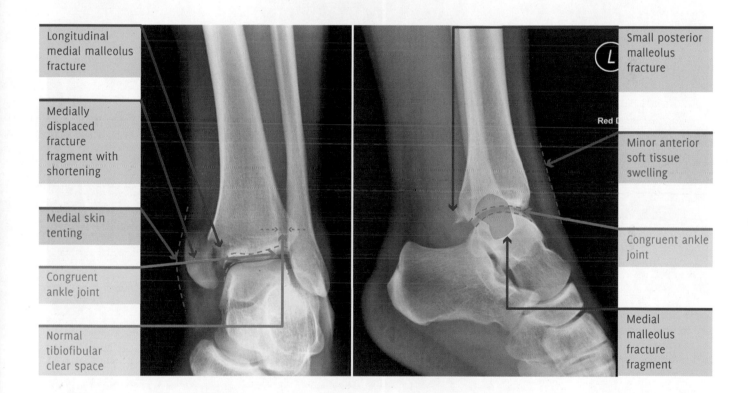

Longitudinal medial malleolus fracture

Medially displaced fracture fragment with shortening

Medial skin tenting

Congruent ankle joint

Normal tibiofibular clear space

Small posterior malleolus fracture

Minor anterior soft tissue swelling

Congruent ankle joint

Medial malleolus fracture fragment

Red D

L

SUMMARY AND DIFFERENTIAL

Both X-rays demonstrate a displaced fracture of the medial malleolus with a small posterior malleolar fracture. There is no talar shift or ankle joint subluxation.

INVESTIGATIONS AND MANAGEMENT

Appropriate analgesia should be provided.

X-rays of the proximal fibula should be reviewed to exclude a Maisonneuve injury.

The ankle should be reduced under sedation in the ED.

A moulded back slab should be applied, and a CT scan performed to check positioning and further delineate the fracture pattern.

A referral should be made to an orthopaedic surgeon who may consider ORIF with medial malleolar screws.

The posterior malleolar fragment appears small and may not require fixation, but this should be considered.

A 46-year-old woman presents to the ED with sudden onset pain over the lateral aspect of her foot and ankle after inverting her ankle while hiking. There is no significant past medical history. On examination, there is no tenderness over the medial and lateral malleoli. The ankle is stable on drawer and stress tests but is tender over the base of the 5th metatarsal and on inversion of foot. She is unable to weight bear. Distal pulses are present. Motor and sensory function is preserved. The injury is closed.

AP mortise and lateral X-rays of the left ankle are requested to assess for fracture.

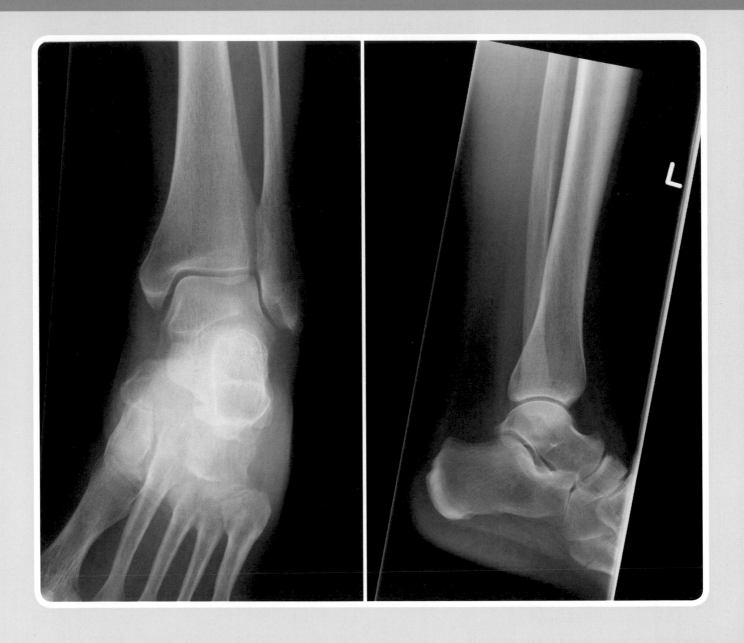

TECHNICAL INFORMATION

Patient ID: Anonymous.
Area: Left ankle.
Projection: AP mortise and lateral.
Technical adequacy:

- Adequate coverage.
- Adequate exposure.
- The patient is not rotated.

● FRACTURE DETAILS

There is an undisplaced fracture involving the base of the 5th metatarsal.

It is difficult to comment on the exact nature of the fracture.

● JOINTS

There is no subluxation or dislocation.

There are no loose bodies.

There is no effusion or lipohaemarthrosis.

There are no arthritic changes.

● SOFT TISSUES

There is no soft tissue swelling.

There is no surgical emphysema.

● BACKGROUND BONE

The background bone is normal.

● BONE LESIONS

There is no bone lesion present.

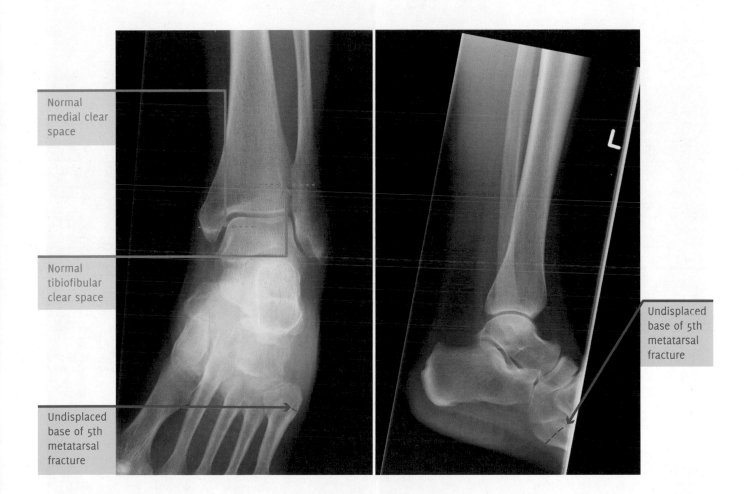

Normal medial clear space

Normal tibiofibular clear space

Undisplaced base of 5th metatarsal fracture

Undisplaced base of 5th metatarsal fracture

SUMMARY AND DIFFERENTIAL

Both X-rays demonstrate an undisplaced fracture at the base of the 5th metatarsal.

INVESTIGATIONS AND MANAGEMENT

Appropriate analgesia should be provided.

Further imaging of the foot (AP, oblique and lateral X-rays) should be obtained to confirm this is a simple base of the 5th metatarsal fracture.

A fixed walking boot should be applied.

The patient should weight bear as pain allows and be referred to the fracture clinic for follow-up.

A 23-year-old woman presents to the foot and ankle clinic with a swelling over the anterolateral aspect of her right ankle. This has been noticeable for some time, but the patient knocked the swelling 2 months ago at which point it became painful. There is no significant past medical history. On examination, there is a smooth firm swelling over the anterolateral aspect of the ankle. It is fixed to the bone. There is no soft tissue tethering. Percussion of the lesion does not produce any neurological symptoms. There is no associated erythema, and the swelling is only mildly tender.

AP mortise and lateral X-rays of the right ankle are requested to assess the swelling.

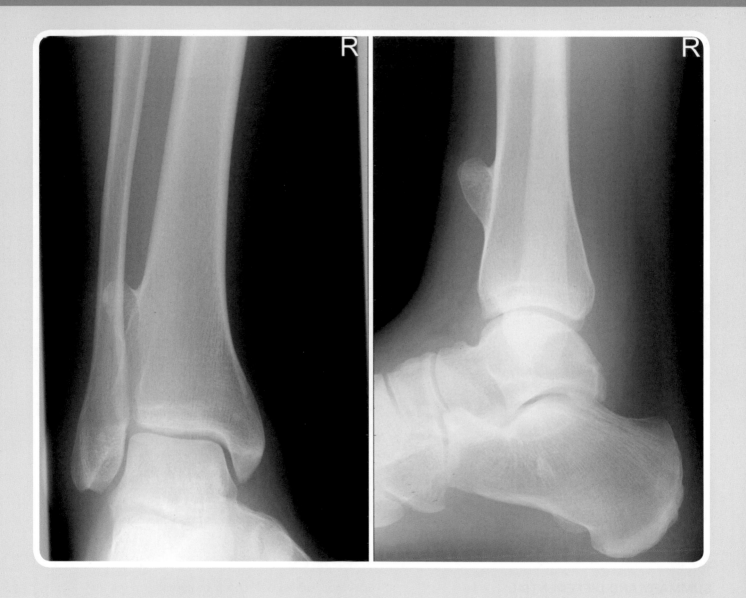

TECHNICAL INFORMATION

Patient ID: Anonymous.
Area: Right ankle.
Projection: AP mortise and lateral.
Technical adequacy:

- Adequate coverage.
- Adequate exposure.
- The patient is not rotated.

● FRACTURE DETAILS

There is no fracture.

● JOINTS

There is no subluxation or dislocation.

There are no loose bodies.

There is no effusion or lipohaemarthrosis.

There are no arthritic changes.

● SOFT TISSUES

There is no soft tissue swelling.

There is no surgical emphysema.

● BACKGROUND BONE

The background bone is normal.

● BONE LESIONS

There is a bone lesion present in the anterolateral cortex of the distal tibia.

The matrix has a trabecular ossified appearance.

It is expansile, exophytic (growing outwards) and pedunculated.

The zone of transition is narrow and well demarcated.

The lesion is in continuity with the metaphysis and extending away from the joint.

There is no bony destruction.

There is no periosteal reaction.

There is no soft tissue mass/component visible.

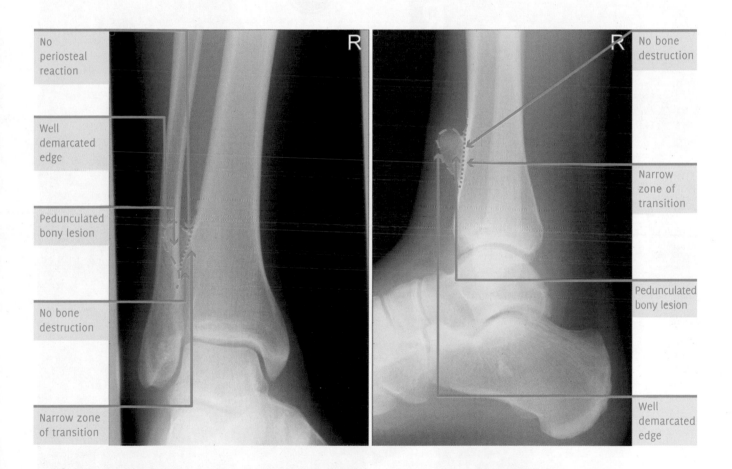

SUMMARY AND DIFFERENTIAL

Both X-rays demonstrate a pedunculated lesion arising from the metaphyseal region of the distal tibia. It is well defined, has a narrow zone of transition and there is no bony destruction. The appearance and description are consistent with an exostosis/osteochondroma of the right tibia. An osteochondroma or exostosis is the most common bone tumour. These lesions, when in isolation, are almost always benign. In inherited conditions such as multiple hereditary exostoses, there is a higher chance of malignant transformation.

INVESTIGATIONS AND MANAGEMENT

Further investigations are not required in general for osteochondromas. If there is growth (after skeletal maturity) or pain, an MRI should be considered to assess for features of malignant transformation.

Treatment is conservative unless the patient is symptomatic. Surgical resection may be considered if the patient is in pain or if there is disruption to surrounding structures, such as nerves or blood vessels. If there is a concern about malignant transformation, then early referral to a bone tumour tertiary centre is recommended.

A 12-year-old girl jumped from her bunk bed landing on her right foot, after which she became unable to weight bear. She is brought to the ED by her parents. There is no significant past medical history. On examination, there is moderate tenderness over the 5th metatarsal. Distal pulses are present. Sensory and motor function is preserved. The injury is closed.

AP and oblique X-rays of the right foot are requested to assess for a fracture.

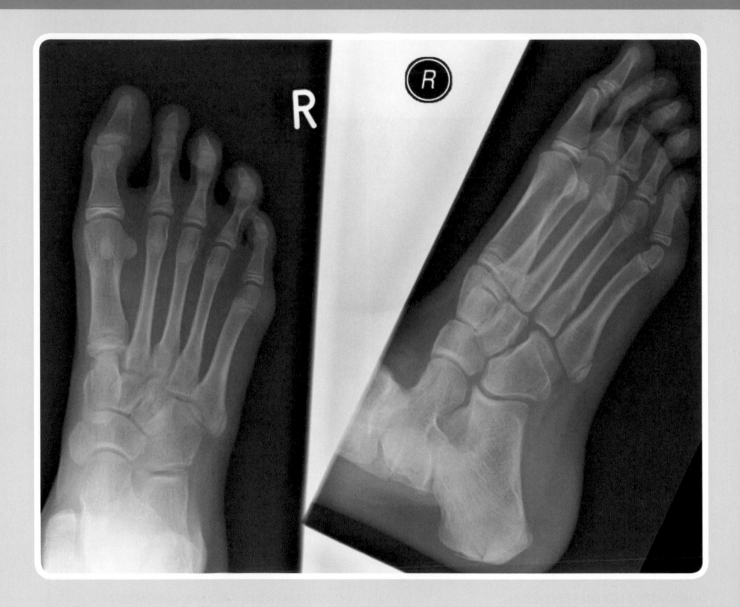

TECHNICAL INFORMATION

Patient ID: Anonymous.
Area: Right foot.
Projection: AP and oblique.
Technical adequacy:

- Adequate coverage.
- Adequate exposure.
- The patient is not rotated.

● FRACTURE DETAILS

There is no fracture.

● JOINTS

There is no subluxation or dislocation.

There are no loose bodies.

There is no effusion or lipohaemarthrosis.

There are no arthritic changes.

● SOFT TISSUES

There is no soft tissue swelling.

There is no surgical emphysema.

● BACKGROUND BONE

The background bone is normal.

● BONE LESIONS

There is no bone lesion present.

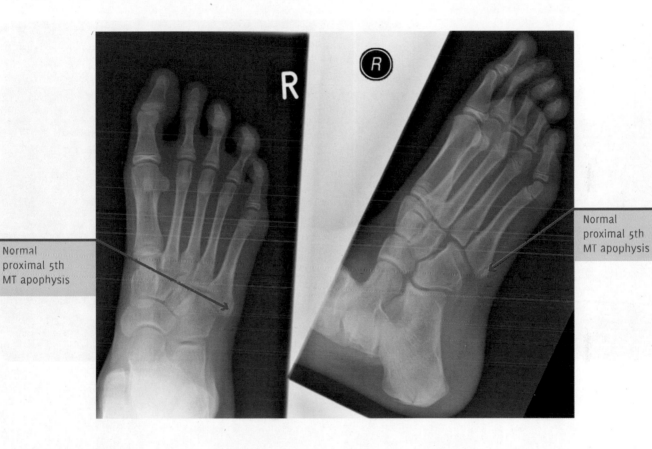

Normal proximal 5th MT apophysis

Normal proximal 5th MT apophysis

SUMMARY AND DIFFERENTIAL

Both X-rays demonstrate a normal paediatric foot X-ray. The appearance at the base of the 5th metatarsal represents the normal proximal 5th metatarsal apophysis.

INVESTIGATIONS AND MANAGEMENT

Appropriate analgesia should be provided.

RICE should be advised, followed by early mobilization.

A 35-year-old burglar jumped from a first storey window during a police chase. He landed on both feet. Subsequently, he has been brought to the ED under police custody. He is unable to weight bear on his left foot. On arrival in the ED, a full ATLS assessment is performed, identifying no immediate life- or limb-threatening injuries. There is no significant past medical history. On examination, the patient is tender over the left heel with significant bruising around the heel and midfoot. Distal pulses are present. Motor and sensory function is preserved. The injury is closed.

Axial and lateral X-rays of the calcaneus are requested to assess for fracture.

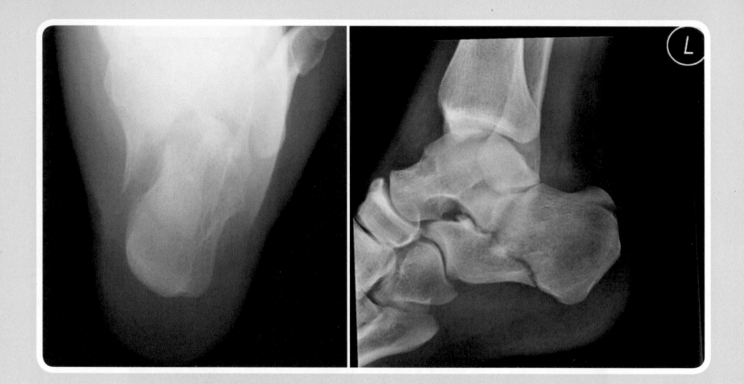

TECHNICAL INFORMATION

Patient ID: Anonymous.
Area: Left calcaneus.
Projection: Axial and lateral.
Technical adequacy:

- Adequate coverage.
- Adequate exposure.
- The patient is not rotated.

● FRACTURE DETAILS

There is a fracture of the calcaneus.

The fracture is oblique, comminuted, intraarticular and involves the subtalar joint.

Displacement is present. Böhler angle is not flattened (>25 degrees).

There is no angulation.

There is no rotation.

There is shortening.

A secondary fracture line is visible exiting the posterior aspect of the calcaneus. This is a minimally displaced tongue type fracture.

It is oblique, simple and intraarticular.

There is no angulation.

There is no rotation.

There is no shortening.

● JOINTS

There is no subluxation or dislocation.

There are no loose bodies.

There is no effusion or lipohaemarthrosis.

There are osteophytes at the talonavicular joint.

● SOFT TISSUES

There is no soft tissue swelling.

There is no surgical emphysema.

● BACKGROUND BONE

The background bone is normal.

● BONE LESIONS

There is no bone lesion present.

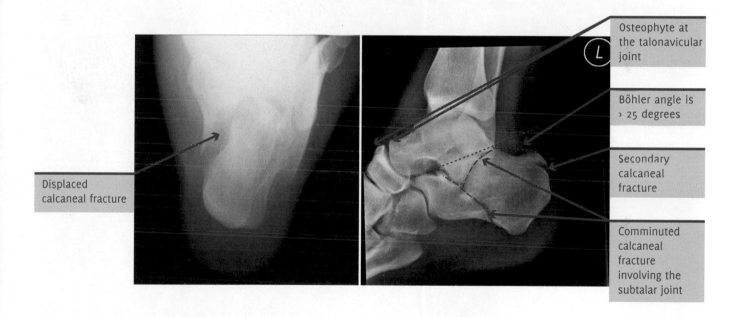

Displaced calcaneal fracture

Osteophyte at the talonavicular joint

Böhler angle is › 25 degrees

Secondary calcaneal fracture

Comminuted calcaneal fracture involving the subtalar joint

SUMMARY AND DIFFERENTIAL

Both X-rays demonstrate an intraarticular calcaneal fracture with a posterior secondary fracture line.

INVESTIGATIONS AND MANAGEMENT

Appropriate analgesia should be provided.

A fall from height such as this should raise alarm for other injuries and the patient should be initially managed as a trauma call with an ATLS protocol. Once life- and immediate limb-threatening injuries have been excluded, a full secondary survey should be performed.

Orthopaedics should be consulted early and the soft tissues around the fracture site inspected. A CT scan is required to further delineate the exact fracture pattern. Surgical intervention for calcaneal fractures may or may not be needed, and an opinion from a foot and ankle trauma surgeon should be sought.

A 24-year-old student has fallen from a horse, twisting her foot in the stirrup. She presents to the ED. There is no significant past medical history. On examination, there is significant swelling and bruising over the right mid- and forefoot. The patient is unable to weight bear because of tenderness over all metatarsal bases. The highest intensity of pain is reported over the 1st metatarsal base. Distal pulses are present. It is not possible to fully assess motor function secondary to pain, but sensation is intact. The injury is closed.

AP, lateral and oblique X-ray views of the right foot are requested to assess for fracture.

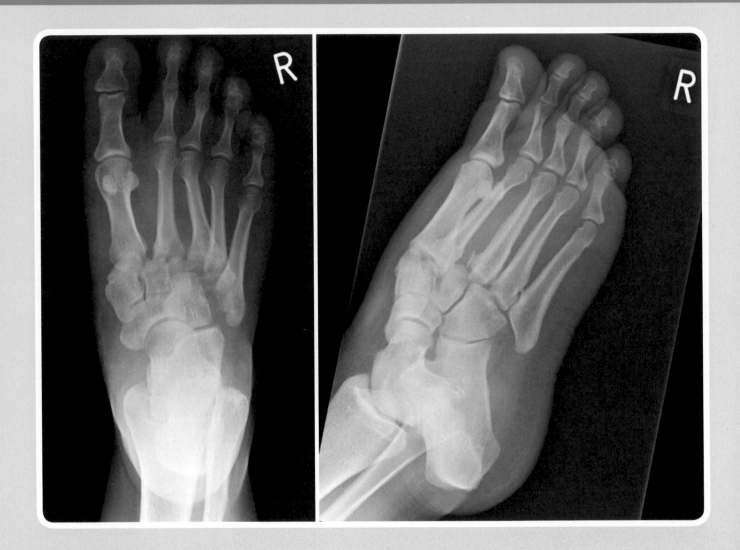

TECHNICAL INFORMATION

Patient ID: Anonymous.
Area: Right foot.
Projection: AP/lateral and oblique.
Technical adequacy:

- Adequate coverage.
- Adequate exposure.
- The patient is not rotated.

● FRACTURE DETAILS

There are fractures involving the 2nd and 3rd metatarsal bases. Further fracture fragments are visible, but their source is not clear on X-ray.

The fractures are oblique, simple and intraarticular.

There is displacement.

There is angulation.

There is rotation.

There is shortening.

● JOINTS

There is lateral subluxation and dislocation of the 1st to 5th tarso-metatarsal joints.

There are no loose bodies.

There is no effusion or lipohaemarthrosis.

There are no arthritic changes.

● SOFT TISSUES

There is soft tissue swelling.

There is no surgical emphysema.

● BACKGROUND BONE

The background bone is normal.

● BONE LESIONS

There is no bone lesion present.

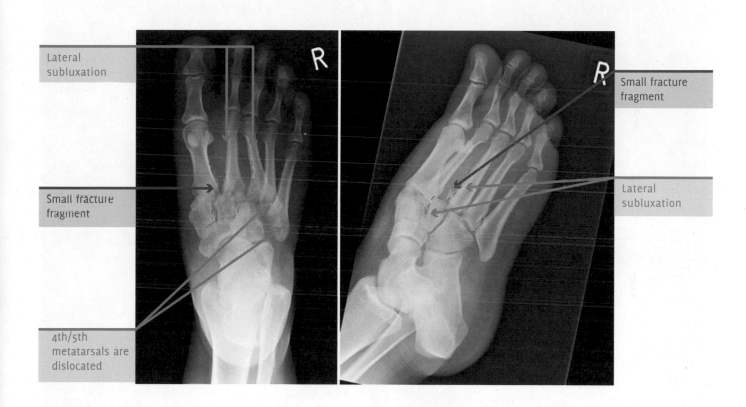

Lateral subluxation

Small fracture fragment

Small fracture fragment

Lateral subluxation

4th/5th metatarsals are dislocated

SUMMARY AND DIFFERENTIAL

Both X-rays demonstrate fractures of the 2nd and 3rd metatarsal bases with lateral subluxation of the 2nd to 5th metatarsals, consistent with a Lisfranc injury.

INVESTIGATIONS AND MANAGEMENT

Appropriate analgesia should be provided.

The limb should be elevated to reduce swelling.

A below-knee back slab or walking boot may be applied to splint the foot.

A referral should be made to an orthopaedic surgeon who may consider ORIF using plate and screw across the Lisfranc ligament complex.

A 28-year-old woman has injured her foot on a cabinet at home and presents to a Minor Injuries Unit. There is no significant past medical history. On examination, there is no significant deformity but there is bruising and pain over the 4th toe and distal metatarsal. She is able to weight bear. The injury is closed.

AP and oblique X-rays of the left foot are requested to assess for fracture.

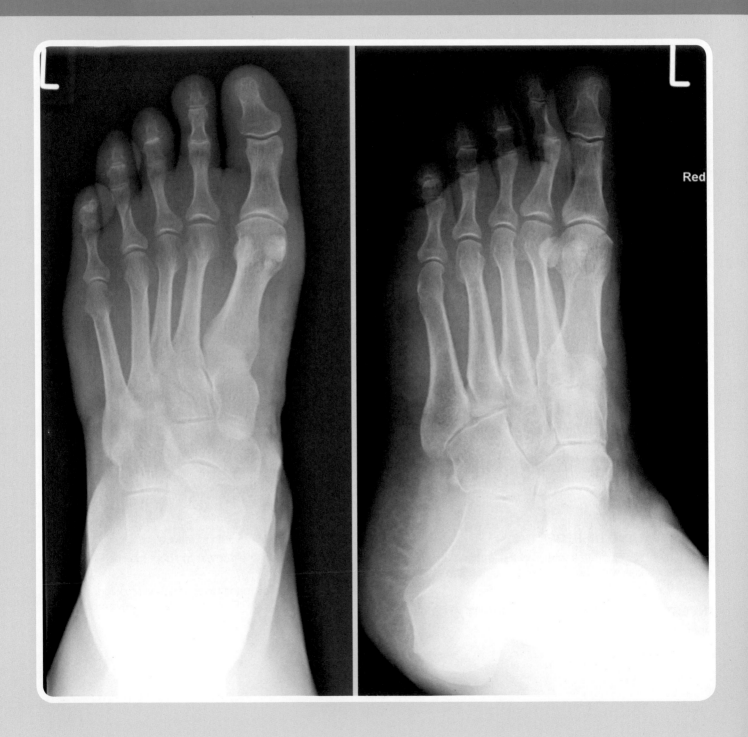

TECHNICAL INFORMATION

Patient ID: Anonymous.
Area: Left foot.
Projection: AP and oblique.
Technical adequacy:

- Adequate coverage.
- Adequate exposure.
- The patient is not rotated.

● FRACTURE DETAILS

There is a fracture involving the proximal phalanx of the 4th toe.

The fracture is spiral, simple and extraarticular.

There is minimal displacement.

There is no angulation.

There is no rotation.

There is no shortening.

● JOINTS

There is no subluxation or dislocation.

There are no loose bodies.

There is no effusion or lipohaemarthrosis.

There are no arthritic changes.

● SOFT TISSUES

There is no soft tissue swelling.

There is no surgical emphysema.

● BACKGROUND BONE

The background bone is normal.

● BONE LESIONS

There is no bone lesion present.

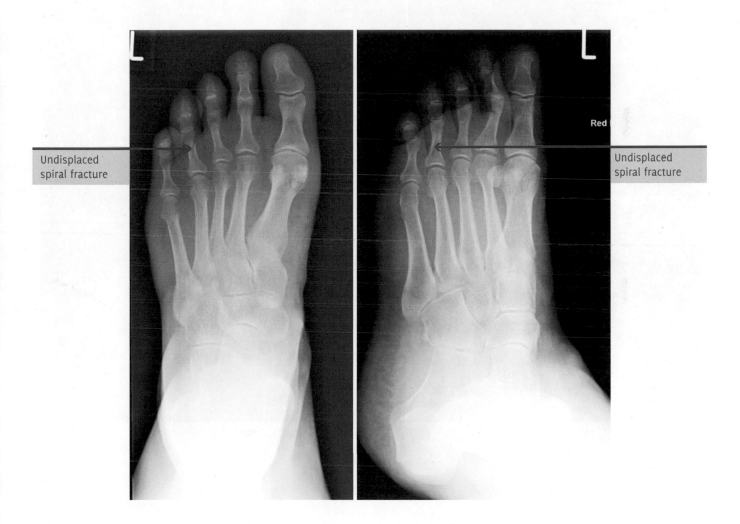

Undisplaced spiral fracture

Undisplaced spiral fracture

Red

SUMMARY AND DIFFERENTIAL

Both X-rays demonstrate a minimally displaced fracture of the proximal phalanx of the 4th toe.

INVESTIGATIONS AND MANAGEMENT

Appropriate analgesia should be provided. A short walking boot should be provided. The patient can weight bear as pain allows and remove the boot when she feels able. A fracture clinic referral should be made.

A 29-year-old semiprofessional football player landed heavily on his left foot after jumping to head the ball. There is no significant past medical history. On examination, there is an obvious varus deformity with skin tenting. He is unable to weight bear. Distal pulses are present on doppler only. There is altered sensation in the foot, and it is not possible to assess motor function secondary to pain. The injury is closed.

AP and lateral X-rays of the left ankle are requested to assess for a fracture.

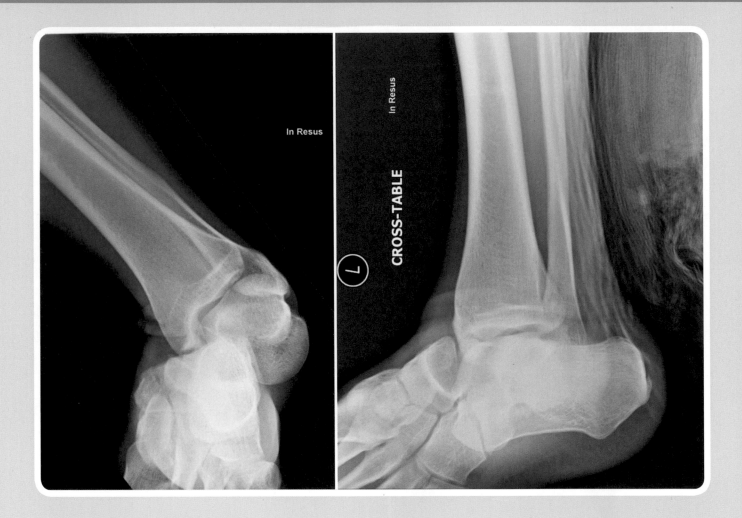

TECHNICAL INFORMATION

Patient ID: Anonymous.
Area: Left ankle.
Projection: AP and lateral.
Technical adequacy:

- Adequate coverage.
- Adequate exposure.
- The patient is not rotated.

● FRACTURE DETAILS

There is no fracture.

● JOINTS

There is dislocation of the talus in relation to the calcaneus and navicular. The distal aspect of the joint is dislocated medially.

The tibiotalar joint and the calcaneocuboid joint remain congruent.

There are no loose bodies.

There is no effusion or lipohaemarthrosis.

There are no arthritic changes.

● SOFT TISSUES

There is tenting of the skin laterally.

There is no surgical emphysema.

● BACKGROUND BONE

The background bone is normal.

● BONE LESIONS

There is no bone lesion present.

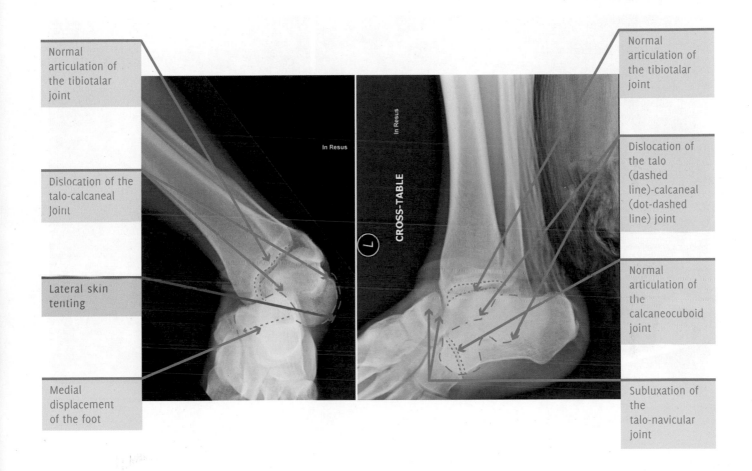

Normal articulation of the tibiotalar joint

Dislocation of the talo-calcaneal joint

Lateral skin tenting

Medial displacement of the foot

Normal articulation of the tibiotalar joint

Dislocation of the talo (dashed line)-calcaneal (dot-dashed line) joint

Normal articulation of the calcaneocuboid joint

Subluxation of the talo-navicular joint

In Resus

CROSS-TABLE

SUMMARY AND DIFFERENTIAL

Both X-rays demonstrate a medial sub-talar dislocation.

INVESTIGATIONS AND MANAGEMENT

Appropriate analgesia should be provided.

The dislocation should be reduced under sedation in the ED with the assistance of orthopaedics as an emergency, as this is a limb-threatening injury.

A moulded back slab should be applied and an X-ray taken to check adequacy of reduction.

A CT should be requested postreduction to assess for associated fractures.

A 42-year-old male, who has a 6-month history of heel pain, attends the fracture clinic. He denies any trauma. There is no significant past medical history. On examination, there is mild tenderness over the heel and focally at the sustentaculum tali. Full range of movement is preserved, and he is able to weight bear.

AP and lateral X-rays of the left calcaneus are requested to assess for a fracture.

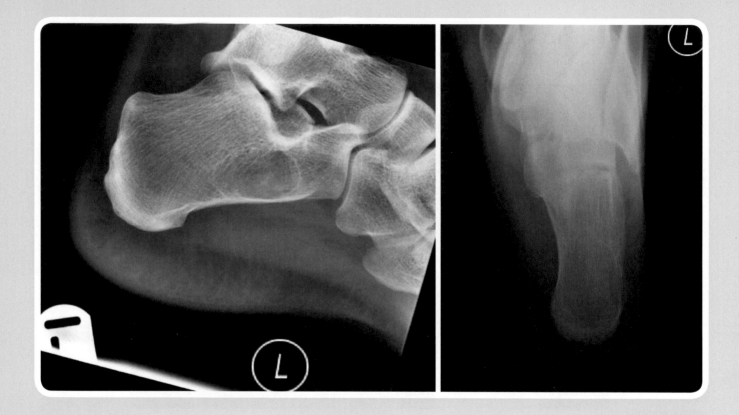

TECHNICAL INFORMATION

Patient ID: Anonymous.
Area: Left calcaneus.
Projection: AP and lateral.
Technical adequacy:

- Adequate coverage.
- Adequate exposure.
- The patient is not rotated.

● FRACTURE DETAILS

There is no fracture.

● JOINTS

There is no subluxation or dislocation.

There are no loose bodies.

There is no effusion or lipohaemarthrosis.

There are no arthritic changes.

● SOFT TISSUES

There is no soft tissue swelling.

There is no surgical emphysema.

● BACKGROUND BONE

The background bone is normal.

● BONE LESIONS

There is a bone lesion present in the medulla that is lucent in appearance but not expansile.

The zone of transition is narrow.

There is no bony destruction.

There is no periosteal reaction.

There is no soft tissue mass/component visible.

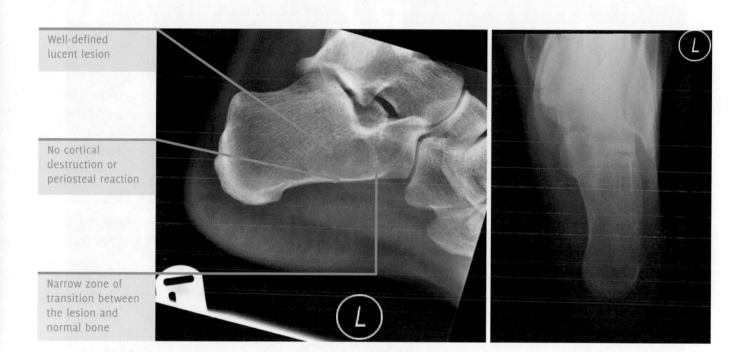

Well-defined lucent lesion

No cortical destruction or periosteal reaction

Narrow zone of transition between the lesion and normal bone

SUMMARY AND DIFFERENTIAL

Both X-rays demonstrate a nonaggressive appearing bone lesion within the calcaneus. Given the location, the findings are consistent with an intraosseous lipoma.

INVESTIGATIONS AND MANAGEMENT

Appropriate analgesia should be provided.

A CT and MRI should be requested to accurately assess the size of the lipoma.

Initial management can be conservative.

If there is ongoing pain, the patient should be referred for consideration of curettage.

A 26-year-old male long-distance runner presents 4 weeks after developing forefoot pain following an ultra-marathon, which has not resolved. There is no significant past medical history. On examination, the patient is tender upon squeezing all MT heads. He is especially tender over the 2nd MT head.

AP and oblique X-rays of the right foot are requested to assess for a fracture.

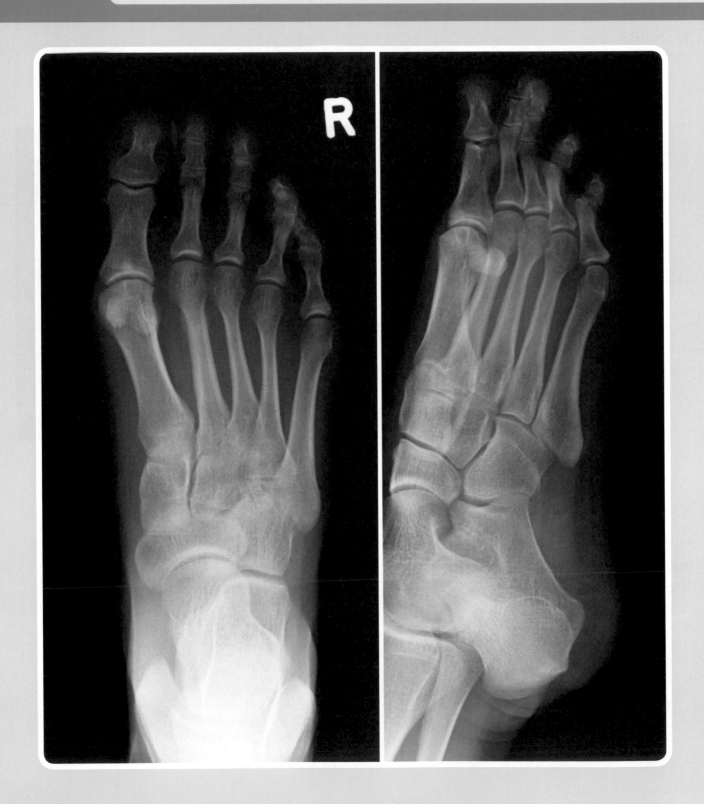

TECHNICAL INFORMATION

Patient ID: Anonymous.
Area: Right foot.
Projection: AP and oblique.
Technical adequacy:

- Adequate coverage.
- Adequate exposure.
- The patient is not rotated.

● FRACTURE DETAILS

There is a periosteal reaction around the neck of the 2nd MT shaft with increased sclerosis in the medulla in this region. This appearance is consistent with a healing stress fracture.

The fracture line is difficult to appreciate but appears simple and extraarticular.

There is no displacement.

There is no angulation.

There is no rotation.

There is no shortening.

● JOINTS

There is no subluxation or dislocation.

There are no loose bodies.

There is no effusion or lipohaemarthrosis.

There are no arthritic changes.

● SOFT TISSUES

There is no soft tissue swelling.

There is no surgical emphysema.

● BACKGROUND BONE

The background bone is normal.

● BONE LESIONS

There is no bone lesion present.

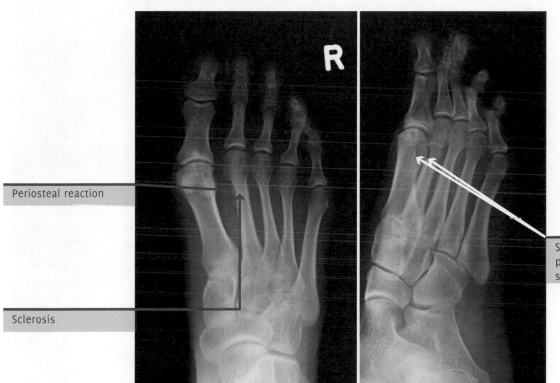

Periosteal reaction

Sclerosis

R

Sesamoid bones projected over the stress fracture site

SUMMARY AND DIFFERENTIAL

Both X-rays demonstrate a periosteal reaction around the distal 2nd MT shaft. Given the location and clinical information, the findings are consistent with a healing stress fracture. No acute fracture is visible.

INVESTIGATIONS AND MANAGEMENT

Appropriate analgesia should be provided.

The patient should be fitted with a fixed walking boot.

Rest and elevation of the foot should be advised.

The patient can weight bear through the foot when wearing the boot, as pain allows.

A referral should be made to the fracture clinic.

A 46-year-old woman presents to the ED with an inversion injury to her left ankle. There is no significant past medical history. On examination, the patient is nontender over the medial and lateral malleoli. The ankle is stable on drawer and stress tests. There is pain over the base of the 5th MT and on eversion of the foot. Distal pulses are present. Sensory and motor function is preserved. The injury is closed.

AP and oblique X-rays of the left foot are requested to assess for a fracture.

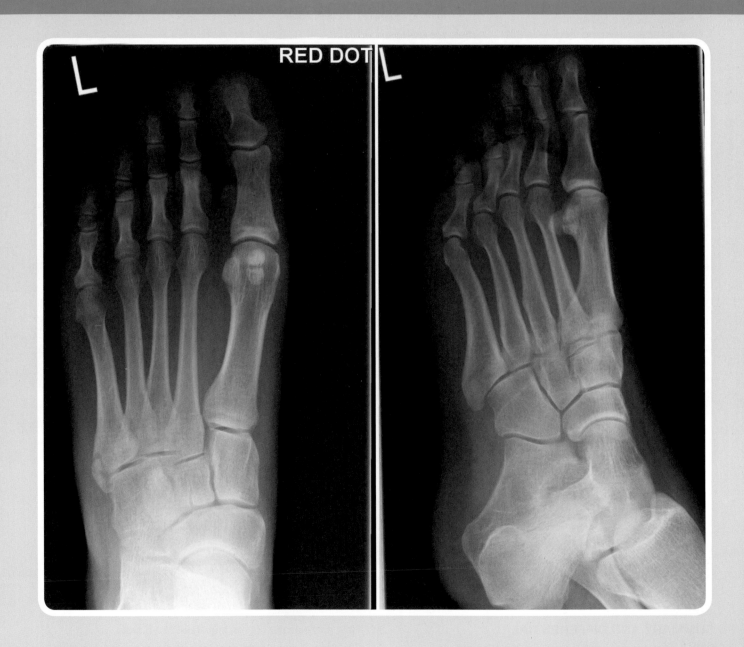

RED DOT

TECHNICAL INFORMATION

Patient ID: Anonymous.
Area: Left foot.
Projection: AP and oblique.
Technical adequacy:

- Adequate coverage.
- Adequate exposure.
- The patient is not rotated.

● FRACTURE DETAILS

There is a fracture involving the 5th MT base.

The fracture is transverse, simple and extraarticular.

Minor lateral displacement is present.

There is no angulation.

There is no rotation.

There is no shortening.

● JOINTS

There is no subluxation or dislocation.

There are no loose bodies.

There is no effusion or lipohaemarthrosis.

There are no arthritic changes.

● SOFT TISSUES

There is no soft tissue swelling.

There is no surgical emphysema.

● BACKGROUND BONE

The background bone is normal.

● BONE LESIONS

There is no bone lesion present.

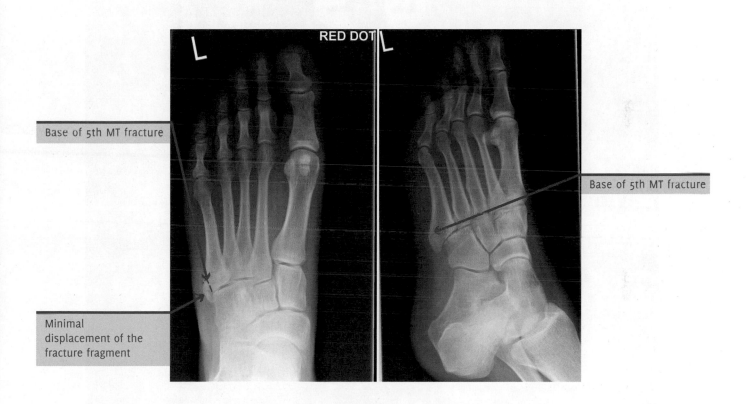

Base of 5th MT fracture

Minimal displacement of the fracture fragment

RED DOT

Base of 5th MT fracture

SUMMARY AND DIFFERENTIAL

These X-rays demonstrate an avulsion fracture at the 5th MT base, with minimal displacement.

INVESTIGATIONS AND MANAGEMENT

Adequate analgesia should be provided.

The patient should be fitted with a fixed walking boot. The patient can weight bear through the foot when wearing the boot, as pain allows.

A referral should be made to the fracture clinic.

A 56-year-old man presents to the ED with a worsening ankle and forefoot deformity on both sides, leading to difficulty fitting into shoes. There is a past medical history of poorly controlled type II diabetes. On examination, there is loss of sensation in a stocking distribution and weak foot pulses. The patient has a grossly deformed left foot and ankle, with significantly reduced range of movement at the ankle and midfoot.

AP and oblique X-rays of the left foot are requested to assess the deformity.

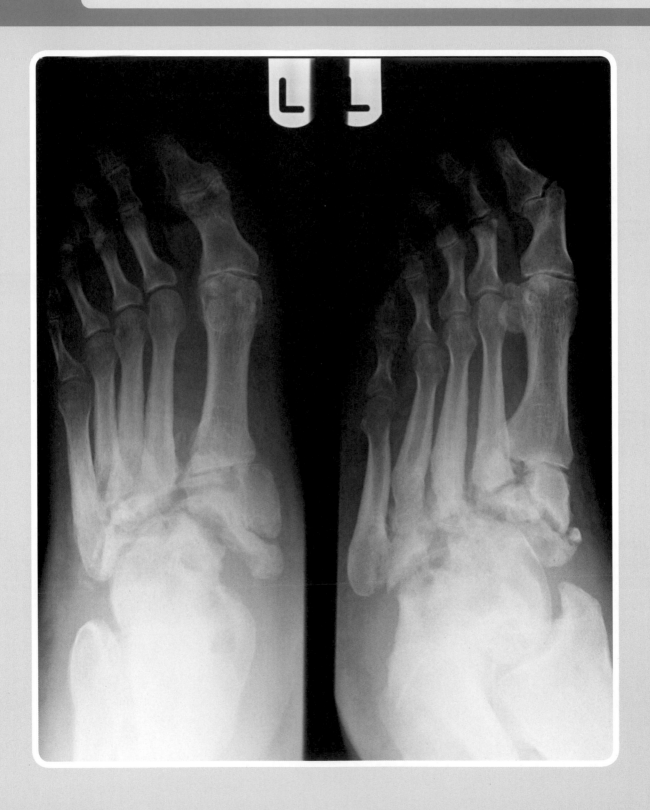

TECHNICAL INFORMATION

Patient ID: Anonymous.
Area: Left foot.
Projection: AP and oblique.
Technical adequacy:

- Adequate coverage.
- Adequate exposure.
- The patient is not rotated.

● FRACTURE DETAILS

There is no fracture.

● JOINTS

The tarsometatarsal joints are grossly abnormal, with marked destructive changes.

There is partial destruction of the cuneiforms, cuboid and navicular, as well as less marked destruction of the metatarsal bases.

Loose bodies are present at the tarsometatarsal joints.

Alignment of the midfoot is difficult to assess because of destruction of the tarsal bones. However, there appears to be lateral subluxation of the 2nd to 5th metatarsals.

There is no effusion or lipohaemarthrosis evident, although this is difficult to assess in the foot on X-rays.

● SOFT TISSUES

There is soft tissue swelling medially.

There is no surgical emphysema.

● BACKGROUND BONE

There is sclerosis of the tarsal and metatarsal bones, in particular of the 2nd and 3rd metatarsals.

● BONE LESIONS

There is no bone lesion present.

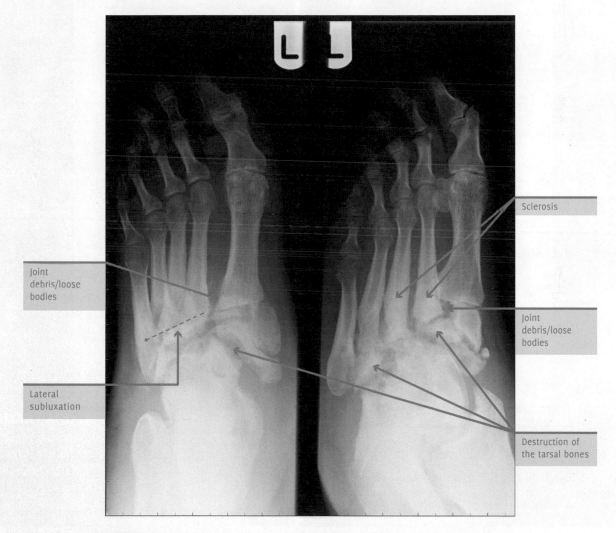

SUMMARY AND DIFFERENTIAL

These X-rays demonstrate grossly deformed tarsometatarsal joints with bony destruction, joint debris (loose bodies), subluxation and increased bone density (sclerosis). The clinical and X-ray findings are consistent with a neuropathic (Charcot) joint.

INVESTIGATIONS AND MANAGEMENT

Appropriate analgesia should be provided.

The patient should be reviewed by a specialist diabetic team for advice about optimization of his diabetic control. A lateral X-ray should be requested to assess for a rocker bottom deformity. The right foot should also be assessed thoroughly.

An urgent referral should be made to orthotics and an orthopaedic surgeon, who may consider total contact casting or surgical intervention.

An 18-year-old female long-distance runner presents with pain over the 2nd and 3rd metatarsals. The pain has worsened over the last few months. There is no significant past medical history. On examination, there is tenderness on squeezing the metatarsals and in particular over the base of the 2nd metatarsal head. Distal pulses are present and sensory and motor function is preserved.

AP and oblique X-rays of the right foot are requested to assess for a fracture.

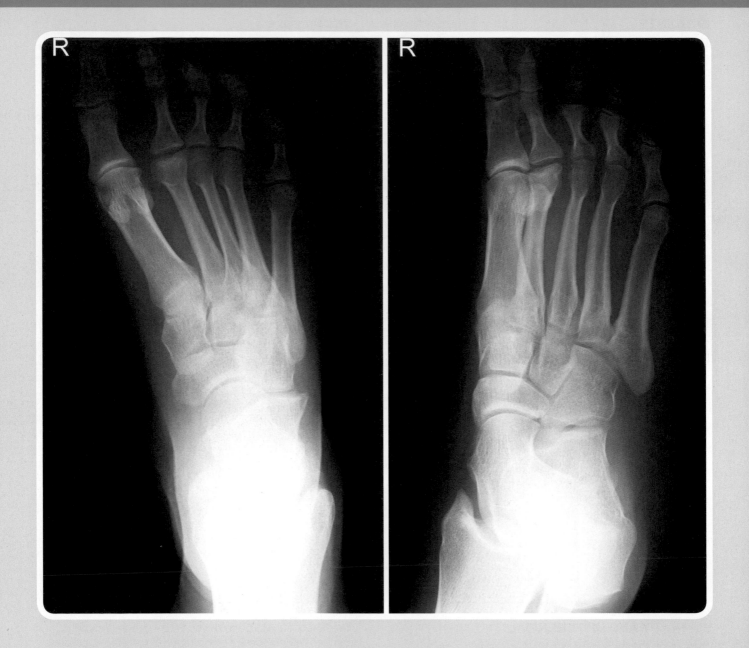

TECHNICAL INFORMATION

Patient ID: Anonymous.
Area: Right foot.
Projection: AP and oblique.
Technical adequacy:

- Adequate coverage.
- Adequate exposure.
- The patient is not rotated.

● FRACTURE DETAILS

There is no acute fracture.

● JOINTS

There is flattening of the 2nd MT head with increased sclerosis and widening of the 2nd MTP joint space.

There is no subluxation or dislocation.

There are no loose bodies.

There is no effusion or lipohaemarthrosis.

There are no arthritic changes.

● SOFT TISSUES

There is no soft tissue swelling.

There is no surgical emphysema.

● BACKGROUND BONE

The background bone is normal.

● BONE LESIONS

There is no bone lesion present.

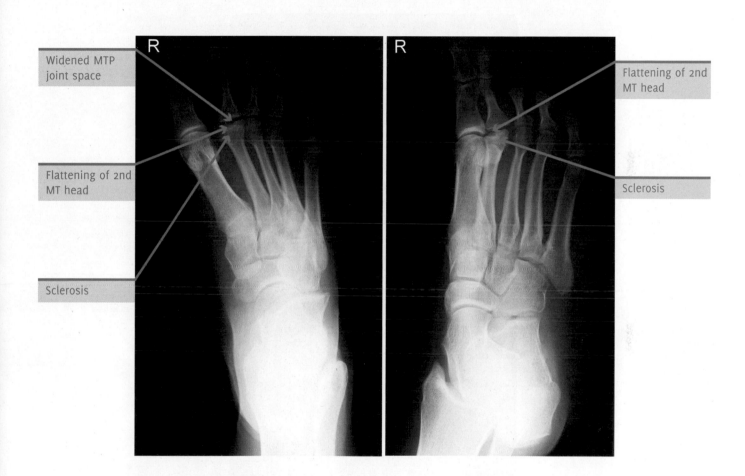

Widened MTP joint space

Flattening of 2nd MT head

Sclerosis

Flattening of 2nd MT head

Sclerosis

SUMMARY AND DIFFERENTIAL

These X-rays demonstrate flattening and sclerosis of the 2nd MT head, consistent with osteochondrosis (Freiburg disease). There is no evidence of MTP osteoarthritis or loose bodies.

INVESTIGATIONS AND MANAGEMENT

Appropriate analgesia should be provided.

The patient should be provided with a walking boot. The patient can weight bear in this as pain allows. She should avoid strenuous activities until the pain has settled. Consider referral to orthopaedics, if symptoms do not settle, for consideration of surgical intervention.

A 63-year-old man who is overweight presents with an acutely painful right great toe. There is no significant past medical history. On examination, the DIPJ of the right great toe is red, hot, inflamed and is exquisitely tender to touch or move. Distal pulses are present and sensory and motor function is preserved.

AP X-rays of the right foot are requested to assess for arthritis.

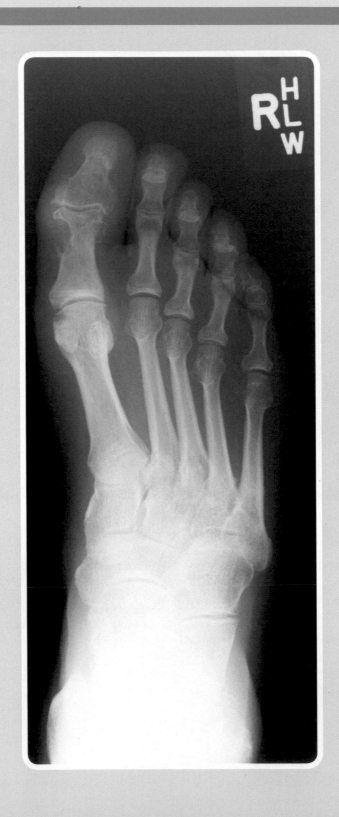

TECHNICAL INFORMATION

Patient ID: Anonymous.
Area: Right foot.
Projection: AP.
Technical adequacy:

- Adequate coverage.
- Adequate exposure.
- The patient is not rotated.

● FRACTURE DETAILS

There is no fracture.

● JOINTS

There is no subluxation or dislocation.

There are no loose bodies.

There is no effusion or lipohaemarthrosis visible.

There are arthritic changes, but the joint spaces are preserved.

● SOFT TISSUES

There is soft tissue swelling medially at the 1st toe IP joint.

There is no surgical emphysema.

● BACKGROUND BONE

The background bone is normal. In particular, there is no periarticular osteopenia.

● BONE LESIONS

There is a well-defined 'punched out' lytic lesion affecting the medial aspect of the proximal phalanx of the 1st toe. Overhanging edges are also visible.

The lesion is adjacent to, but separate from, the 1st IP joint.

There is no soft tissue mass or component visible.

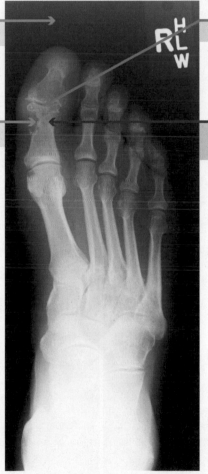

Overhanging edge

Preserved joint space

"Punched-out" lesion

Normal mineralization of bone – no periarticular osteopenia

SUMMARY AND DIFFERENTIAL

These X-rays demonstrate a well-defined juxtaarticular lytic lesion affecting the proximal phalanx of the 1st toe. The adjacent bone and IP joint space are normal. The findings are consistent with gout in the DIPJ of the great toe.

INVESTIGATIONS AND MANAGEMENT

Adequate analgesia should be provided.

FBC and CRP should be performed to assess for possible septic arthritis or osteomyelitis and a referral made to orthopaedics if there are any concerns.

Depending on renal function, the patient should be prescribed NSAIDs and/or colchicine in the acute phase and allopurinol should be considered for future prophylaxis.

A 62-year-old with known foot pressure ulcers presents with increasing left foot pain and a raised temperature. There is a past medical history of type II diabetes and previous vascular surgery on the left foot. On examination, there are deep ulcers over the balls of both feet. There is cellulitis surrounding the ulceration and tenderness is elicited over the 4th MT of the left foot. Distal pulses are not palpable and are monophasic on doppler. There is a loss of sensation in a stocking distribution.

AP and oblique X-rays of the left foot are requested to assess for possible osteomyelitis.

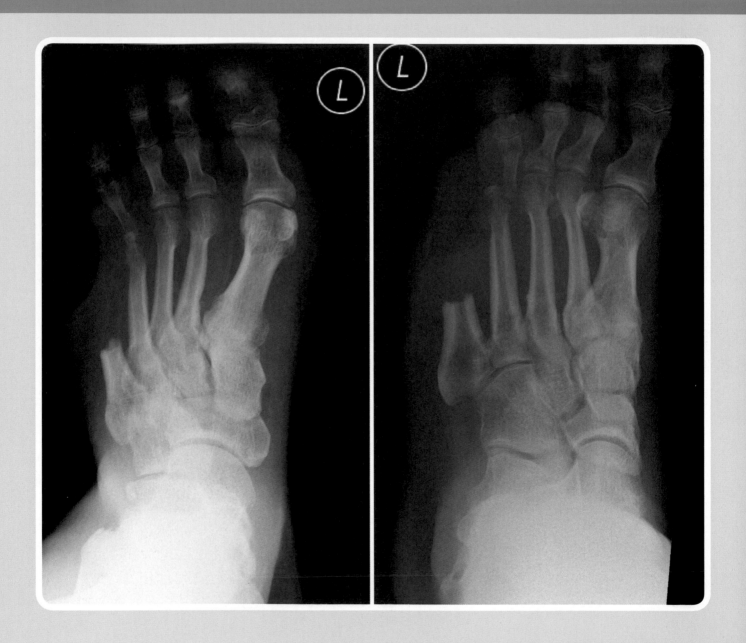

TECHNICAL INFORMATION

Patient ID: Anonymous.
Area: Left foot.
Projection: AP and oblique.
Technical adequacy:

- Adequate coverage.
- Adequate exposure.
- The patient is not rotated.

FRACTURE DETAILS

There is no fracture.

JOINTS

There is subluxation of the 4th MTP joint, best seen on the oblique view.

There are no loose bodies.

There is no effusion or lipohaemarthrosis.

There are no arthritic changes.

SOFT TISSUES

There is no soft tissue swelling.

There is no surgical emphysema.

Vascular calcification is present.

BACKGROUND BONE

There is osteopenia in the proximal phalanx of the 4th toe.

The remaining background bone is normal.

BONE LESIONS

There is a previous amputation of the 5th MT shaft and head, and the 5th toe.

There is ill-defined bone destruction of the 4th MT head and base of the proximal phalanx of the 4th toe. The bone destruction involves articular and nonarticular surfaces.

There is no soft tissue mass or component visible.

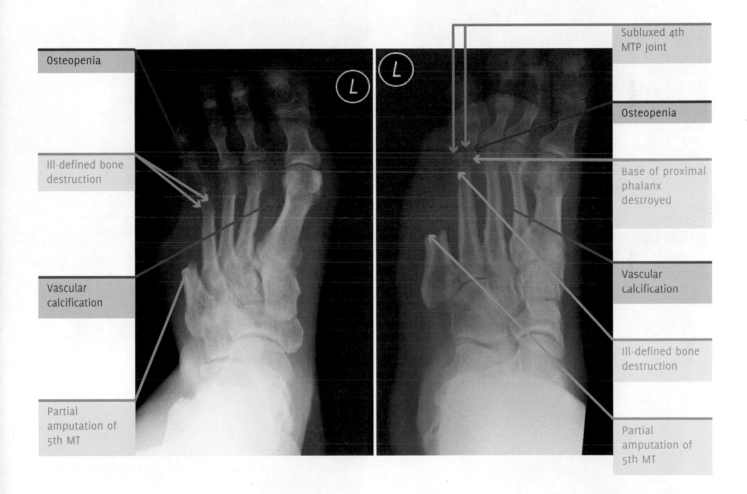

Osteopenia

Ill-defined bone destruction

Vascular calcification

Partial amputation of 5th MT

Subluxed 4th MTP joint

Osteopenia

Base of proximal phalanx destroyed

Vascular calcification

Ill-defined bone destruction

Partial amputation of 5th MT

SUMMARY AND DIFFERENTIAL

These X-rays demonstrate destructive lesions involving the 4th MTP joint. Given the past history and clinical findings, the appearances are consistent with osteomyelitis.

INVESTIGATIONS AND MANAGEMENT

Adequate analgesia should be provided.

The patient should be prescribed appropriate IV antibiotics, guided by local policy and culture results.

A referral should be made to a diabetic foot MDT.

If ulceration and tissue damage are severe, the patient may require an amputation.

A 12-year-old boy was helping his father with some gardening when a large stone fell onto his great toe. He is brought to the ED complaining of pain and a swollen great toe. There is no significant past medical history. On examination, the great toe is swollen and tender. Movements of the toe exacerbate the pain. Distal pulses are present and sensory and motor function is preserved. The injury is closed.

AP and oblique X-rays of the right great toe are requested to assess for a fracture.

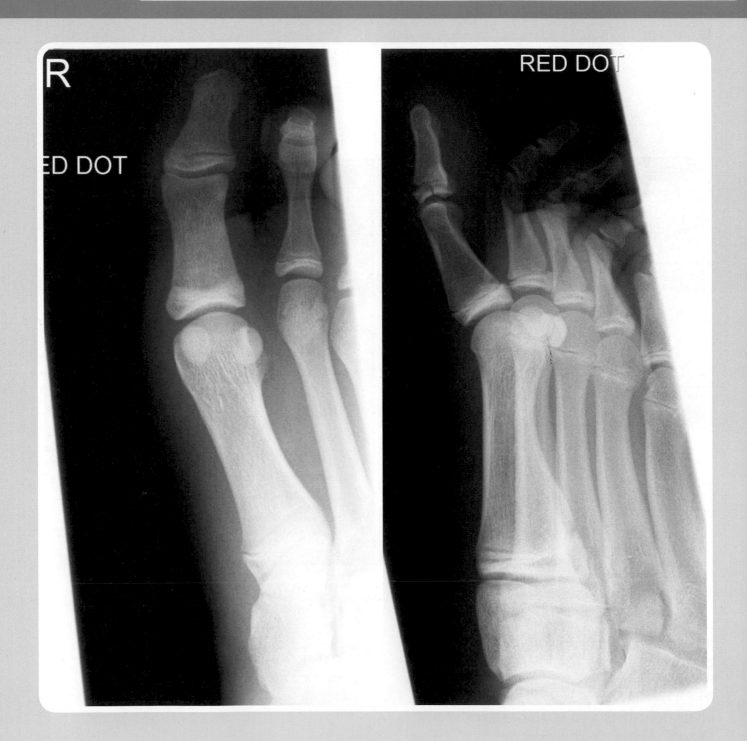

TECHNICAL INFORMATION

Patient ID: Anonymous.
Area: Right great toe.
Projection: AP and oblique.
Technical adequacy:

- Adequate coverage.
- Adequate exposure.
- The patient is not rotated.

● FRACTURE DETAILS

There is a fracture of the distal phalanx of the great toe, involving the epiphysis and physis.

The fracture is transverse, simple and intraarticular.

There is no displacement, although the physis appears widened superiorly.

There is no angulation.

There is no rotation.

There is no shortening.

● JOINTS

There is no subluxation or dislocation.

There are no loose bodies.

There is no effusion or lipohaemarthrosis.

There are no arthritic changes.

● SOFT TISSUES

There is soft tissue swelling present around the great toe.

There is no surgical emphysema.

● BACKGROUND BONE

The background bone is normal.

● BONE LESIONS

There is no bone lesion present.

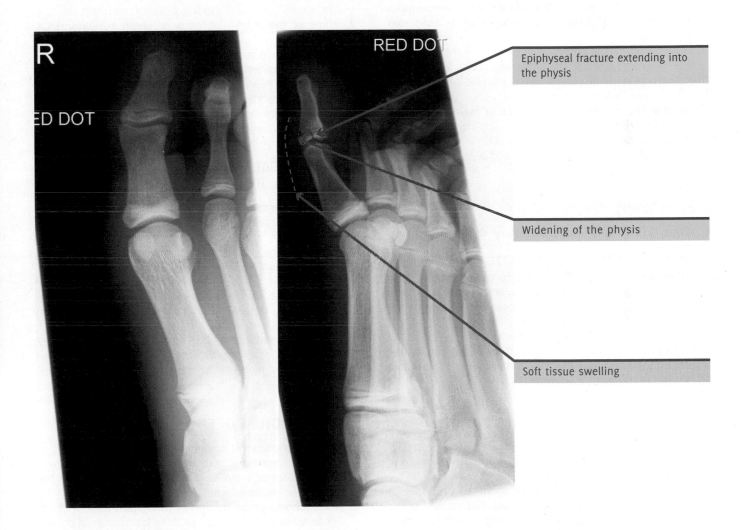

Epiphyseal fracture extending into the physis

Widening of the physis

Soft tissue swelling

SUMMARY AND DIFFERENTIAL

Both X-rays demonstrate a minimally displaced fracture of the distal phalanx of the great toe. The fracture involves the physis and epiphysis, consistent with a Salter-Harris Type 3 fracture.

INVESTIGATIONS AND MANAGEMENT

Advice regarding analgesia should be provided.

The patient can wear a fixed walking boot for 2 to 4 weeks for pain relief, and can weight bear fully as pain allows.

Referral should be made to fracture clinic.

Case Questions and Answers

CASE 1: SCAPHOID WAIST FRACTURE

1. **Where does the main blood supply to the scaphoid come from?**
   The main blood supply enters the scaphoid distally and there is retrograde blood flow towards the proximal pole.
2. **Where on the hand will the patient have tenderness if there is a suspicion of an underlying scaphoid fracture?**
   Patients report pain and have tenderness in the ASB. This is an area on the radial side of the wrist that is identified by extending the thumb. The ASB can then be found radial to the extensor pollicis longus tendon.
3. **What is the correct initial treatment for a suspected scaphoid fracture?**
   Suspected scaphoid fractures should be immobilized in a temporary wrist or scaphoid cast and a referral made to orthopaedics.

CASE 2: BENNET'S FRACTURE

1. **What is the mechanism of injury that causes this fracture?**
   An axial load on the thumb with it held in a flexed position.
2. **What are the different directions of movement can occur at the thumb (carpo-metacarpal) joint?**
   The thumb has a wide range of movement. The directions of movement possible are flexion, extension, abduction, adduction, circumduction and opposition.
3. **What is a common long-term effect of leaving a displaced intraarticular fracture to heal with a malunion (healed in the wrong position)?**
   Secondary arthritis leading to pain and loss of function.

CASE 3: MALLET FRACTURE

1. **What structure is attached to the dorsal fragment that is avulsed in a mallet fracture?**
   The extensor tendon to the finger attaches to the dorsal surface of the distal phalanx. It is avulsed leading to an inability to extend the finger. This gives the characteristic mallet appearance.
2. **What are the indications for surgical fixation for this fracture?**
   Subluxation of the joint and a fracture fragment that involves >50% of the articular surface.
3. **If the fracture is left and the patient develops arthritis later, what would be the appropriate treatment?**
   Arthritis of the distal interphalangeal joint is best treated with fusion.

CASE 4: PROXIMAL PHALANX AVULSION FRACTURE

1. **Which structure of the thumb metacarpophalangeal joint stabilizes the joint during pinch grip?**
   The ulnar collateral ligament (UCL) is important in hand function as it stabilizes the finger during pinch grip.
2. **What is the name commonly given to ulnar UCL injuries?**
   UCL injuries are sometimes called *skier's thumb*.
3. **What is a Stener lesion?**
   A Stener lesion is where the avulsed ligament, either with or without a bony fragment, displaces superficial to the adductor aponeurosis and therefore will not be able to heal without surgical intervention.

CASE 5: DORSAL DISLOCATION OF CARPO-METACARPAL JOINTS

1. **What percentage of carpal metacarpal joint (CMCJ) dislocations are missed on initial assessment?**
   Up to 25% of these injuries are missed, especially if a true lateral radiograph of the hand is not requested.
2. **How are these fractures best managed?**
   The dislocated CMCJ's need to be reduced and held with K wires. There are often associated fractures and occasionally, open reduction and internal fixation is required to restore articular congruity.
3. **If missed, what is the long-term impact of this injury?**
   This injury leads to a reduction in power grip. If there is an associated intraarticular fracture, then secondary arthritis can occur.

CASE 6: FRACTURE OF ENCHONDROMA

1. **Where are enchondromas most commonly found?**
   The most common location is the hand followed by feet, then distal femur, proximal humerus and then tibia. It is the most common bone tumour in the hand.
2. **Are enchondromas benign or malignant tumours?**
   These are benign tumours, but there is a very small chance of malignant transformation. More commonly in the hand, they can cause a problem when a fracture occurs through the lesions.
3. **Why is it important to differentiate between a solitary enchondroma and multiple enchondromas?**
   Patients with multiple enchondromas are at a higher risk of one of the tumours becoming malignant. They also may be at risk of developing other malignancies and should undergo surveillance.

CASE 7: BUCKLE FRACTURE OF RADIUS

1. What is a buckle fracture?

This is an incomplete fracture of a paediatric bone where one cortex is intact, and the other has undergone plastic deformation and 'buckled'.

2. What complication can occur when there is a paediatric fracture at a growth plate?

A growth arrest may occur. This could be partial or complete and can lead to shortening or a deformity of a limb if the growth stops. It is important to understand which fractures are particularly associated with a growth arrest.

3. How are growth plate fractures classified?

The Salter-Harris classification is used for growth plate injuries. There are five types of fracture. The higher the number, the higher the risk of growth arrest.

CASE 8: DISTAL RADIUS FRACTURE

1. Which two joints are present at the distal radius?

The two joints are the distal radial joint, which is an articulation between the radius and scaphoid/lunate, and the distal radioulnar joint.

2. How is a buckle fracture of the distal radius best treated?

A buckle fracture of the distal radius is best treated in a splint for 3 weeks to allow symptom relief followed by mobilization.

3. What movement occurs at the distal radioulnar joint?

Pronation and supination occur at both the proximal and distal radioulnar joints. In supination, the palm is facing up and in pronation the palm is facing down.

CASE 9: DISTAL RADIUS AND ULNAR FRACTURES

1. Where in the hand do you test for sensory function of the median nerve?

The radial border of the index finger.

2. Is the anterior interosseus nerve (AIN) likely to be injured in this fracture?

No, the AIN can be injured in paediatric supracondylar fractures but not in distal radius fractures.

3. Is it likely a growth arrest would occur as a result of this injury?

The fracture does not involve the growth plate so it is unlikely a growth arrest would occur. However, if treated with manipulation and K wires, there could be iatrogenic damage to the growth plate leading to a growth arrest.

CASE 10: DISTAL RADIUS BUCKLE FRACTURE

1. At what age do growth plates fuse and bones stop growing?

The exact time varies based on the bone, the sex of the patient and the onset of menarche. As a basic rule, girls stop growing around age 14 years, or 2 years after menarche, and boys stop growing aged 16 years.

2. Where does the majority of growth occur in the arm?

In the arm, most growth occurs at the proximal humerus and the distal radius. It is important to know this as the more active growth plates have a higher ability to remodel but also the impact of a growth arrest will be more severe.

3. Name the proximal row of carpal bones from the radial to ulnar side of the wrist.

Scaphoid, lunate, triquetrum, pisiform.

CASE 11: INTRAARTICULAR RADIUS FRACTURE AND ULNAR STYLOID FRACTURE

1. How is shortening of the radius measured on an X-ray?

Radial shortening is best assessed through ulnar variance. This is the difference between the height of the radius and the ulnar. Normally, the radius is slightly higher or prominent at the wrist than the ulnar but if there is shortening, the radius will be shorter than the ulnar on the X-ray.

2. What is the normal amount of volar tilt in the distal radius?

Volar tilt is measured on the lateral X-ray and refers to the normal angulation of the distal radius. Normally there is around 10 degrees of volar angulation.

3. What is radial inclination?

This is a measure of how prominent the radial styloid is on the AP X-ray. It is measured as an angle between the flat articular surface of the distal radius and the tip of the styloid. Measurements are useful to understand how displaced a distal radius fracture is and may help decide on what surgery if any is needed.

CASE 12: INTRAARTICULAR RADIUS FRACTURE AND ULNAR FRACTURE

1. What is the definition of a Smiths fracture?

A Smith's fracture is a volarly angulated or displaced extraarticular fracture of the distal radius.

2. Why are these fractures more commonly treated with surgery than dorsally angulated fractures?

It is more difficult to reduce and hold these fractures by manipulation under anaesthetic. Even if an initial reduction is achieved, they tend to redisplace and therefore generally should all at least be considered for operative intervention.

3. This patient presents with pins and needles in the thumb and index finger at the same time as this fracture. What complication has occurred because of the injury?

The patient has symptoms of carpal tunnel syndrome. This can occur because of the fracture and the associated swelling. It can also occur if a fracture is reduced and held in a cast with a lot of flexion and ulnar deviation at the wrist.

CASE 13: DISTAL RADIUS AND ULNAR FRACTURES

1. What does the term carpal malalignment mean?

This refers to whether the carpal bones of the hand are aligned with the radial shaft on a lateral radiograph. In this case they clearly are not.

2. An inadequate reduction is achieved, and the surgeon decides on surgery. What operation is recommended in this patient?

Given the degree of displacement, it is unlikely a closed reduction could be achieved and then held with K wires. Therefore the surgical preference would be open reduction and internal fixation through the volar surface of the forearm.

3. What muscle/tendon extends the thumb?

Extensor pollicis longus. This tendon can sometimes rupture as a result of a wrist fracture, so it is important to test for thumb extension in patients who have broken their wrist.

CASE 14: DISTAL RADIUS AND ULNAR METAPHYSEAL FRACTURES

1. In this case, the patient presents without a radial pulse. Why does the hand remain pink despite this loss of pulse?

The hand receives its blood supply from both the ulnar and radial arteries. The arteries join via anastomoses in the hand. Therefore despite occlusion of the radial artery perfusion to the hand can remain.

2. What measures can be taken in the emergency department to reduce pain from this fracture?

Simple analgesia should always be prescribed as a baseline. However, the most effective way to improve pain is to perform a provisional reduction and apply a temporary cast, which can splint the fracture.

3. The child develops significant swelling and uncontrolled pain out of proportion with what is normal. What complication has occurred?

This clinical picture is in keeping with compartment syndrome. The pressure from the swelling is too high, causing muscle damage. If a patient develops this, they need surgery as an emergency to release the pressure.

CASE 15: INTRAARTICULAR DISTAL RADIUS FRACTURE

1. What is the definition of a volar Barton's fracture?

This is a partial articular fracture of the distal radius where there is a volar intraarticular fragment that is displaced volarly. The dorsal cortex and articular surface are intact.

2. In a younger, more active patient, how would this fracture be treated?

This fracture is best treated with open reduction and internal fixation with the aim to buttress the volar fragment back up against the intact dorsal cortex. This can be achieved with volar plate fixation.

3. The patient develops stiffness, cold and hot intolerance, skin discolouration and severe pain in the weeks following surgery. What complication has occurred because of the injury?

This could be a case of complex regional pain syndrome. The patient requires hand therapy and hand physiotherapy to improve movement as well as desensitization to reduce pain.

CASE 16: COLLES FRACTURE

1. Is there carpal malalignment in this fracture?

Yes. On the lateral X-ray, there is dorsal angulation, which leads to the line drawn along the carpal bones to be dorsal to the shaft of the radius.

2. How much dorsal angulation is there?

There is 30 to 40 degrees of dorsal angulation (10 degrees of volar angulation is normal).

3. What type of cast will be applied when this fracture is reduced and why?

Wrist fractures are often treated initially with a temporary cast. This goes halfway around the wrist, is held in place with a bandage and can be changed to a full cast later. The temporary cast can stabilize the fracture and provide pain relief but also allows space for swelling to occur as is often the case in the first few days following the injury.

CASE 17: DISTAL RADIUS FRACTURE WITH TERRY THOMAS SIGN

1. What structure is injured in a scapholunate dissociation?

The scapholunate ligament is ruptured. This ligament is crucial in ensuring the proximal carpal bones move and function normally.

2. What early problems could the patient develop as a result of this injury?

Patients with an untreated or missed scapholunate injury may initially present with pain on the dorsum and radial side of the wrist. They may also report mechanical type symptoms such as clicking or catching.

3. What are the late complications of this injury?

If left untreated, the patient will continue to have abnormal movements in the wrist. Over time this leads to arthritis in a predictable fashion and is given the term *scapholunate advanced collapse* (*SLAC* wrist).

CASE 18: TRANS-SCAPHOID PERILUNATE DISLOCATION WITH ASSOCIATED RADIAL STYLOID FRACTURE

1. What is the difference between a perilunate and a lunate dislocation?

In a perilunate dislocation, the lunate remains in its anatomical position, but the capitate is dislocated dorsally. In a lunate dislocation, the lunate is dislocated volarly.

2. What structures are contained within the carpal tunnel?

The four tendons of flexor digitorum superficialis, the four tendons of flexor digitorum profundus, flexor pollicis longus and the median nerve.

3. What are the boundaries of the carpal tunnel?

The roof of the tunnel is the flexor retinaculum, the floor is the carpal bones, the ulnar border is the hamate and the radial border is the trapezium.

CASE 19: INTRAARTICULAR DISTAL RADIUS FRACTURE

1. What complication can occur because of a displaced intraarticular fracture?

If left malreduced, then the forces through the joint are abnormal and this could lead to secondary arthritis.

2. Why do intraarticular fractures have a higher rate of nonunion?

When a fracture is intraarticular, synovial fluid may escape into the fracture line and stop or slow a fracture from healing. Intraarticular fractures also tend to be higher energy, which means there may be more soft tissue disruption including to the blood supply to the bone.

3. **What bony prominence can be felt on the dorsal aspect of the wrist?**

Lister's tubercle. This bony prominence is a useful landmark for identifying where the wrist joint is. If the tubercle is palpated and the examiner moves distally, they will find a soft spot, which is where the wrist joint can be found.

CASE 20: TRIQUETRAL FRACTURE

1. **What more serious fracture/dislocation are triquetral fractures associated with?**

While the vast majority of triquetral fractures are simple and can be treated nonoperatively, they can occasionally be associated with a perilunate/lunate fracture dislocation.

2. **What is the likely mechanism of injury that has caused this fracture?**

This is an avulsion fracture where dorsal ligaments have been avulsed from the triquetrum together with a small amount of bone.

3. **What articulates with the volar surface of the triquetrum?**

The pisiform. The triquetrum and pisiform form the pisotriquetral joint, which can occasionally develop arthritis and become painful.

CASE 21: GALLEAZZI FRACTURE-DISLOCATION

1. **What is meant by the term a fracture of necessity?**

A fracture of necessity is one that must be treated surgically to avoid a poor outcome.

2. **What is the surgical treatment for this fracture?**

The radius needs to be anatomically reduced and help with open reduction and internal fixation.

3. **What associated fracture indicated possible distal radioulnar joint (DRUJ) instability?**

If there is an associated ulnar styloid fracture, there is a higher chance that the DRUJ will remain unstable.

CASE 22: RADIUS AND ULNA SHAFT FRACTURES

1. **What structure surrounds the diaphysis of bones and provides a blood supply to the bone?**

The periosteum is a complex layer of tissue that surrounds the shaft of bones and provides a blood supply. It is a thick easily identifiable structure in children but by the time people are elderly it is hardly visible.

2. **The fracture is manipulated into an acceptable position and held with a cast. How high up the forearm or arm should the cast go?**

Forearm fractures need to be casted above the elbow to prevent rotational movements in the forearm, which could lead to fracture displacement.

3. **What structure should be protected when inserting flexible nails in children to prevent a long-term complication?**

Flexible intramedullary nails are inserted into the bone just proximal or distal to the growth plate to avoid damage to this structure and a future growth arrest.

CASE 23: RADIUS AND ULNA SHAFT FRACTURES

1. **What is the relevance of the thick paediatric periosteum in the management of paediatric forearm fractures?**

Sometimes the bone can fracture without rupturing the periosteum. This periosteum provides a degree of support and can help maintain the reduction of a fracture together with an appropriate cast. This means many paediatric fractures can be treated with less surgery than the equivalent fracture in adults.

2. **What nerve is at risk of injury during insertion of the radial flexible nail from just proximal to the radial styloid?**

The superficial radial nerve is near the insertion point, and this must be protected during surgery.

3. **Why is bone age important when considering how to manage paediatric fractures?**

Paediatric bones can remodel. The amount of potential to remodel depends on the location of the fracture relative to where the bone is growing most and how much growth is left.

CASE 24: MONTEGGIA FRACTURE-DISLOCATION

1. **What is required to allow the radial head to reduce from its dislocated position in this injury?**

If the fracture can be reduced into an anatomical position by closed reduction/manipulation, then the radial head will often reduce from its dislocated position.

2. **If the radial head will not reduce despite achieving the above, what may be blocking reduction?**

The annular ligament surrounds the radial head and can become entrapped in the joint when the radial head dislocates. This then blocks reduction even if the ulnar is reduced.

3. **What muscles originate from the medial epicondyle of the humerus?**

This is the site of the common flexor origin. Pronator teres, flexor carpi radialis, palmaris longus, flexor digitorum superficialis and flexor carpi ulnaris originate here.

CASE 25: INTRAARTICULAR OLECRANON FRACTURE

1. **What tendon attaches to the olecranon?**

The triceps tendon attaches at the olecranon.

2. **What is the function of this tendon?**

It facilitates the triceps muscle extending the elbow.

3. **How is the function of this tendon best checked on examination?**

Extension of the elbow must be examined for in a way whereby gravity has been eliminated. The best way to achieve this is to abduct the shoulder and with the forearm pronated ask the patient to extend their elbow out to the side.

CASE 26: DISTAL HUMERUS FRACTURE WITH ASSOCIATED ELBOW SUBLUXATION

1. **What structure passes around the medial epicondyle of the humerus?**

   The ulnar nerve passes through the interosseus membrane proximal to the elbow joint and passes posterior to the medial epicondyle.

2. **What is the motor branch of the median nerve that arises just distal to the elbow joint and what does it supply?**

   The anterior interosseus nerve. This nerve supplies pronator quadratus, flexor pollicis longus and the radial half of flexor digitorum profundus.

3. **What nerve innervates the triceps?**

   The radial nerve innervates triceps, which functions to extend the elbow.

CASE 27: RADIAL NECK FRACTURE

1. **Why is it better to treat this patient in a sling rather than a cast?**

   A sling provides adequate support while allowing gentle mobilization as pain allows. This undisplaced fracture is very unlikely to displace but patients can develop stiffness. A cast could worsen that stiffness and should be avoided if possible, particularly around the elbow.

2. **What movement might the patient report does not return fully to normal despite physiotherapy?**

   While the radial head is involved in rotational movement at the radiocapitellar joint, this fracture is more commonly associated with a loss of full extension at the elbow. However, because the shoulder and hands are mobile, the impact of a small amount of fixed flexion deformity is negligible.

3. **What two other bones does the radial head articulate with?**

   The radial head articulates with the ulnar at the proximal radioulnar joint and with the capitellum of the distal humerus as a part of the elbow joint.

CASE 28: RADIAL NECK SALTER-HARRIS TYPE 2 FRACTURE

1. **What is the correct treatment for this fracture?**

   While this fracture is displaced, the overall alignment is good and therefore this could be treated for 4 weeks in a cast or just in a sling.

2. **If the fracture was more displaced how could this be treated surgically?**

   The fracture could first be reduced with manipulation and direct pressure over the radial neck. If the fracture reduces and is stable, it could be held in a cast. If unstable or is not reducing, then percutaneous reduction and/or fixation can be attempted.

3. **What nerve is very close to the radial neck and if injured, how would this present?**

   The posterior interosseus nerve wraps around the radial head/neck. This nerve supplies the extensors of the wrist and if injured, will present in a patient with a wrist drop.

CASE 29: GARTLAND TYPE 2 SUPRACONDYLAR FRACTURE

1. **If left malreduced, what deformity will be visible in the arm?**

   Supracondylar fractures, which heal with a malunion, typically develop a cubitus varus deformity (gunstock deformity), which, while cosmetically unappealing, generally have a good functional outcome.

2. **What structure is at risk when placing a percutaneous wire from the medial side of the elbow?**

   The ulnar nerve is at risk when placing wires from the medial side. For this reason, if a wire is to be placed from this side, then the ulnar nerve should be visualized and protected.

3. **What is the large tendon that is palpable in the antecubital fossa when the elbow is flexed?**

   This is the tendon of biceps brachii. It is innervated by the musculocutaneous nerve and is a flexor of the elbow.

CASE 30: HUMERUS SPIRAL FRACTURE

1. **The patient develops a wrist drop after the application of a cast. What structure has been injured?**

   The radial nerve can become entrapped in fractures at this level, and this causes a wrist drop.

2. **If the above happens, what is the next correct clinical step?**

   If a wrist drop occurs after cast application with this fracture, then exploration of the fracture and surgical fixation is required. The radial nerve is explored and removed from the fracture and the fracture fixed with a plate at the same time.

3. **Why might it be advantageous to surgically fix this fracture rather than an above elbow cast?**

   Fixation of the fracture would allow earlier mobilization as no splint across the elbow would be required. A long-arm cast could lead to long-term stiffness at the elbow joint but does avoid the need for surgery.

CASE 31: NECK OF HUMERUS FRACTURE WITH ANTERIOR DISPLACEMENT

1. **Should this patient be given a collar and cuff or a broad-arm sling?**

   A collar and cuff are best for proximal humerus fractures with the elbow flexed and the hand held high and close to the chest. This allows the elbow to be free and under the influence of gravity, which supports reduction of the fracture.

2. **What large muscle is innervated by the axillary nerve, attaches to the humerus and abducts the shoulder?**

   This is the deltoid muscle. It forms the contour of the shoulder and is a strong abductor. This muscle is used as a landmark together with pectoralis major to approach the shoulder joint surgically.

3. **What structure attaches to the great and lesser tuberosities of the proximal humerus?**

   The rotator cuff muscles attach to the tuberosities and have many key roles in shoulder function.

CASE 32: POSTERIOR SHOULDER DISLOCATION (PREVIOUS STABILIZATION SURGERY)

1. Apart from seizure, what other mechanism of injury is associated with posterior shoulder dislocations?

Electrocution is also associated with this type of dislocation although it is extremely rare.

2. What position will the arm be held in when the shoulder is dislocated posteriorly?

The arm is held in internal rotation when dislocated posteriorly. Any attempts to externally rotate are extremely painful.

3. What large shoulder muscle that abducts the shoulder does the axillary nerve supply?

The axillary nerve supplies the deltoid muscle.

CASE 33: COMMINUTED PROXIMAL HUMERUS FRACTURE AND DISLOCATION

1. What structures are at risk of injury from the fractured end of the shaft of the humerus in this fracture?

The shaft of the humerus is sitting in the axilla. The brachial plexus and axillary artery are both at risk of injury although these complications are rare.

2. What are the two most proximal bony fragments seen in the X-ray?

The two most proximal bony fragments represent the greater and lesser tuberosity.

3. What structures attach to the greater and lesser tuberosity?

The rotator cuff attaches to these two bony prominences of the shoulder. Supraspinatus, infraspinatus and teres minor attach to the greater tuberosity and subscapularis attaches to the less tuberosity.

CASE 34: ANTERIOR SHOULDER DISLOCATION

1. How is axillary nerve function clinically assessed?

Sensation is tested over the regimental badge patch area and motor function is assessed by testing for shoulder abduction.

2. What is a Bankart lesion?

This is a tear of the anterior glenoid that has occurred because of an anterior dislocation. It can be associated with an avulsion fracture, and this is called a *bony Bankart lesion*.

3. What is a Hill-Sachs lesion?

This is an impaction fracture of the humeral head that occurs at the time of an anterior dislocation. If the area of impaction is large, there is a higher risk of further dislocations.

CASE 35: ANTERIOR SHOULDER DISLOCATION

1. What is the most common technique used to reduce anterior shoulder dislocations?

The most common and safest way is to apply traction to the arm with the arm in an abducted position. A co-worker needs to apply counter traction often with a sheet under the axilla. This is a safe approach if done gradually with sedation.

2. What clinical features would be found on examination if there is a torn rotator cuff?

There are many special tests for shoulder examination. The rotator cuff initiates abduction and provides internal and external rotation. Therefore these movements will be weak. The special tests such as the drop arm test assess for this.

3. Which rotator cuff muscle is responsible for initiating abduction at the shoulder?

Supraspinatus initiates abduction and then continues to assist deltoid in abduction.

CASE 36: CALCIFIC TENDONITIS

1. What is the initial treatment of choice for a patient presenting with this condition and shoulder pain to their primary care physician?

The majority of the time this painful condition resolves with time, NSAIDs, rest and physiotherapy.

2. Which tendon is involved in this case?

The supraspinatus tendon is affected.

3. If initial treatments do not work, what alternative options are available?

If initial treatments are not effective, then steroid injections can help. If not, there are more invasive options including ultrasound guided needle lavage, needle barbotage, subacromial decompression and extracorporeal shockwave therapy.

CASE 37: PNEUMOTHORAX

1. Given the mechanism of injury, what is the most likely cause of the pneumothorax?

There is most likely an underlying rib fracture, which has damaged the pleura leading to the pneumothorax.

2. What imaging could be obtained in the ED resus room to better understand the extent of the chest injury?

A chest X-ray would be a simple way to radiologically assess the chest injury. Depending on the extent of suspected injuries, a CT scan might also be helpful.

3. The surgeons decide a chest drain is needed. What structure is at risk of injury if the drain is inserted too low on the right side of the chest?

Chest drains need to be inserted in the 5th intercostal space just anterior to the mid-axillary line. If inserted too low, then the liver is at risk on the right side and the spleen on the left.

CASE 38: ACROMIOCLAVICULAR JOINT INJURY

1. What classification system is used for this injury?

The Rockwood classification describes both the severity of injury and guides the potential need for surgery. Type 1–3 dislocations, where the distal clavicle is <100% dislocated, can be treated without surgery. Type 4–6 dislocations are more severe and require surgery.

2. What ligaments are likely torn as a result of this injury?

The coracoclavicular ligaments are torn. These ligaments run from the coracoid to the clavicle and hold the clavicle in its usual anatomical position.

3. What functional impairment will occur if this injury is left untreated?

Secondary acromioclavicular joint arthritis may cause pain towards the end range of abduction of the shoulder. So, this could impair above head activities.

CASE 39: ACROMIOCLAVICULAR JOINT DISLOCATION

1. What is the function of the clavicle?

The clavicle functions to hold the shoulder girdle away from the axial skeleton and allows the shoulder and arm to function. It also provides protection to important neurovascular structures including the subclavian vein and the brachial plexus.

2. What structure sits under the acromion and above the rotator cuff?

The subacromial bursa sits between the acromion and the rotator cuff. This can become inflamed, and this is called a *subacromial bursitis*.

3. What is the treatment for secondary ACJ arthritis?

The first line of treatment is to use analgesia, physiotherapy and injections. If these nonoperative measures do not work, then arthroscopic excision of the ACJ can be performed.

CASE 40: COMMINUTED MID-CLAVICULAR FRACTURE

1. What is the nonunion rate for clavicle fractures?

Approximately 10% of clavicle fractures go on form to a nonunion. Not all of these nonunions (where the bone has not healed) are symptomatic, but a small number of patients with clavicle fractures require fixation after a period of nonoperative treatment.

2. If surgical fixation is attempted what structures are at risk?

There are superficial sensory nerves, which can be damaged during the surgical approach. This can lead to localized loss of sensation and occasionally neuroma formation. The subclavian vein, artery and the brachial plexus are very close to the surgical field and very rarely can be damaged. This can lead to significant life-threatening bleeding although this is very rare.

3. Name two muscles that attach or originate from the clavicle?

The sternocleidomastoid muscle attaches to the clavicle. The deltoid muscle has a wide origin that includes the clavicle and the acromion.

CASE 41: FRACTURE OF DISTAL THIRD OF CLAVICLE

1. What bone does the distal clavicle articulate with?

The distal clavicle articulates with the acromion. This is a bony prominence of the scapula. This articulation is the acromioclavicular joint.

2. What is the nonunion rate for distal clavicle fractures?

There is a higher nonunion rate in distal clavicle fractures compared to midshaft fractures. Displaced fractures have up to a 50% nonunion rate and require surgical fixation. If the fracture is minimally displaced as in this case, then nonoperative treatment will likely be successful.

3. What are the surgical options for fixation of these fractures?

There are several options for fixation although fixation with a plate is the most used technique.

CASE 42: WEDGE FRACTURES AND SUPERIOR ENDPLATE FRACTURE

1. What imaging modality is used to assess for osteoporosis?

A DEXA scan assesses for bone density. DEXA stands for Dual Energy X-ray Absorptiometry. The machine assesses how much the bone absorbs X-rays and this is compared to expected bone density absorption rates.

2. If an elderly patient develops a compression fracture without trauma, what condition needs to considered?

Metastatic cancer needs to be considered in patients presenting with atraumatic spinal fractures.

3. If the patient has ongoing pain despite nonoperative measures what surgical option can provide pain relief?

Vertebroplasty can be performed. Under X-ray guidance, a cannulated needle is inserted into the vertebral body and cement injected to stabilize the vertebra. Balloon kyphoplasty can also be attempted, whereby the collapse of the vertebra is corrected to an extent through balloon dilatation and then cement injected into the space.

CASE 43: UNILATERAL SACROILIITIS

1. What are the differential diagnoses for a unilateral sacroiliitis?

The differentials include infection, ankylosing spondylitis, Reiter syndrome and osteoarthritis.

2. What further imaging is required to assess for infection?

An MRI scan will demonstrate inflammation at the sacroiliac joint and will also demonstrate if there is an associated abscess that needs drained.

3. What blood tests should the patient undergo?

Infection/inflammatory markers such as CRP, white cell count and erythrocyte sedimentation rate are helpful. HLA B-27 should be taken if ankylosing spondylitis is suspected. Blood cultures should also be performed.

CASE 44: UNILATERAL FACET JOINT DISLOCATION

1. What is the imaging modality of choice to assess for a spinal fracture in a stable polytrauma patient?

A CT scan will most accurately assess the cervical spine. X-rays increasingly have less of a role, partly because it can be difficult to adequately assess the entirety of the cervical spine for C1-T1.

2. Which X-ray view is required to assess for a C1/C2 injury?

An open mouth odontoid peg view will demonstrate any fracture of the odontoid peg but will also demonstrate the relationship between the lateral masses of C1 and C2. If there is an increased distance between the lateral mass of C1 and the odontoid peg, then there is potentially an unstable ligamentous injury affecting C1/C2.

3. **What is the eponymous name given to the burst fracture of C1/atlas?**

This is called the *Jeffersons fracture* and occurs when an axial force is applied to the head. This is often seen in people who dive into shallow water.

CASE 45: BILATERAL SYMMETRICAL SACROILIITIS

1. **What are the clinical features of ankylosing spondylitis?**

Patients are normally young to middle aged adults and present with gradual worsening lumbar pain and early morning stiffness with insidious onset. They may also present with hip or pelvic pain and stiffness. Neck pain and deformity with an increasing inability to look forward is generally a later clinical feature.

2. **What other conditions are associated with ankylosing spondylitis?**

Ankylosing spondylitis is associated with anterior uveitis, cardiac disease, pulmonary fibrosis and renal amyloidosis.

3. **What is the first-line treatment of choice for patients with ankylosing spondylitis?**

Simple treatments such as NSAIDs and physiotherapy are the first-line treatments. Biological agents like TNF-alpha blocker such as Etanercept may also be considered.

CASE 46: EXTRACAPSULAR NECK OF FEMUR FRACTURE

1. **What is the maximum amount of time that a patient should wait between hip fracture and surgery?**

Studies show that patient mortality increases if hip fracture patients wait longer than 36 hours following injury. Surgery should therefore only be delayed if there is a modifiable medical condition and the patient's fitness for surgery can be improved.

2. **What factors impact mortality in hip fracture patients?**

Patients with hip fractures need MDT care with preoperative optimization with input from orthogeriatrics and good postoperative care. The choice of surgical operation and the timing of that surgery also impacts on mortality rates.

3. **Why are extracapsular fractures treated with fixation rather than a replacement arthroplasty?**

In extracapsular fractures, the blood supply is preserved to the femoral head. There is therefore a low risk of secondary avascular necrosis. With appropriate surgical fixation where the fracture is reduced and stabilized with either a dynamic hip screw or an intramedullary nail the fracture should go on to heal.

CASE 47: SUBTROCHANTERIC FEMORAL FRACTURE

1. **What conditions can cause a pathological subtrochanteric fracture?**

The list includes metastatic cancer, primary bone tumours (malignant or benign), bisphosphonate use and osteoporosis.

2. **What is the surgical treatment of choice for this fracture?**

This fracture is best treated surgically with a long intramedullary nail extending from the greater trochanter down to the distal femoral metaphysis.

3. **What complication is this fracture predisposed to following surgical fixation?**

This fracture has a high rate of nonunion despite adequate surgical fixation. This can present with late implant failure where the intramedullary nail breaks and requires further fixation.

CASE 48: ANTERIOR DISLOCATION OF TOTAL HIP REPLACEMENT

1. **Which surgical approach for total hip replacement (THR) is associated with a higher dislocation rate?**

The posterior approach is often quoted as being associated with a higher dislocation rate. In part, this is caused by historical techniques whereas the dislocation rates with a modern surgical technique are far lower than in the past.

2. **What are the potential causes for the lucent line around the acetabular component?**

The lucent line represents either aseptic or septic loosening. Therefore periprosthetic joint infection should be considered. Otherwise, over time hip replacement components can become loose.

3. **What would the treatment be if the patient has had multiple dislocations and is fit for further surgery?**

Revision hip surgery, where the old implants are removed and new ones inserted, can be performed.

CASE 49: PERIPROSTHETIC FEMORAL SHAFT FRACTURE

1. **What different fixation techniques can be used to stabilize a hip replacement device within the bone?**

Hip replacement components can either be fixed within the bone using cement or using an uncemented implant, which has a porous lining that encourages bone fixation through ingrowth.

2. **What preoperative factors should be considered before surgery?**

This patient is elderly, has had a previous hip fracture and has vascular calcification. This would suggest they potentially are medically frail and should have their medical health optimized before surgery.

3. **Which fixation technique is associated with a higher periprosthetic fracture rate in the early postoperative period?**

Uncemented femoral components, which need a tight 'press' fit within the bone have a higher rate of intraoperative or early fracture. However, cemented implants have a higher rate of late periprosthetic fracture.

CASE 50: OSTEOARTHRITIS OF THE HIP

1. **What are the radiological features of osteoarthritis?**

Radiological features include subchondral sclerosis, subchondral cysts, osteophytes and loss of joint space.

2. **How would a patient with hip arthritis present?**

Patients typically present with pain in the groin, anterior thigh and lateral thigh, stiffness, an antalgic gait, and difficulty with day-to-day activities such as washing, dressing, putting on shoes or getting into and out of cars. Occasionally, hip arthritis can present with knee pain, which can cause confusion for the clinician.

3. How effective is total hip replacement surgery as a treatment for advanced hip arthritis?

Hip replacement surgery is one of the most effective operations across all specialties for improving quality of life. Ninety-five percent of patients are satisfied with the result of their surgery and for many, the operation represents a new lease of life.

CASE 51: INTERTROCHANTERIC NECK OF FEMUR FRACTURE

1. How does a dynamic hip screw work?

A dynamic hip screw is made up of a large screw that fits inside the barrel of a plate. The screw is inserted into the femoral head and the plate fixed to the lateral cortex. As the patient begins to weight bear after surgery the screw slides, but cannot rotate, inside the barrel of the plate. This allows compression at the fracture site. This stabilizes the fracture, encourages bone healing and allows patients to mobilize with less pain.

2. The patient develops a fever and shortness of breath 3 days postop. What is the most likely diagnosis?

Pneumonia is very common in patients presenting with a hip fracture. Clinicians should have a low index of suspicion for chest infection and ensure antibiotics are commenced early.

3. The patient develops sudden onset chest pain 2 weeks after surgery with a sinus tachycardia on their ECG and hypoxia despite 15-L oxygen. What is the most concerning diagnosis?

Pulmonary emboli are rare but potentially life threatening. Thrombolysis is not possible because of recent surgery.

CASE 52: CANNULATED HIP SCREWS FROM PREVIOUS FRACTURE

1. What is the blood supply to the femoral head?

The femoral head received the majority of its blood supply from the anterior and posterior circumflex femoral arteries, which form an anastomosis around the femoral neck. In children, there is additional blood supply from the artery of ligamentum teres.

2. What are the surgical options for intracapsular fractures?

The surgical options include fixation with either screws or a dynamic hip screw, or a hip replacement, which can either be a hemiarthroplasty or a total hip replacement.

3. What complication can occur when an intracapsular fracture is treated with surgical fixation?

In an intracapsular fracture, there is a high chance with fixation that the fracture does not heal, and the patient develops avascular necrosis.

CASE 53: CEMENTED HEMIARTHROPLASTY

1. What is the difference between a total hip replacement and a hemiarthroplasty?

In a total hip replacement, the acetabulum, femoral neck and femoral head are replaced. In a hemiarthroplasty, the acetabulum is not replaced.

2. What surgical approach is commonly used for inserting a hemiarthroplasty in patients with a hip fracture?

A lateral approach is most used (although this does vary in different countries). This has a lower rate of dislocation than other approaches.

3. What serious but rare cement-related complication can occur during or shortly after surgery?

Rarely, patients can develop a cement implantation reaction. There is a sudden drop in blood pressure and hypoxia. This can be fatal. Overall, the mortality rate is lower if cemented hemiarthroplasty implants are used rather than uncemented equivalents.

CASE 54: UNCEMENTED HEMIARTHROPLASTY

1. What anatomical structures attach to the greater trochanter?

The main structures attaching to the greater trochanter are the gluteus medius and minimus. These two muscles abduct the hip.

2. What was the likely reason this implant was used for this patients' previous hip fracture?

This is an uncemented implant, which can be implanted quickly. Given the patients frailty, it is likely that the anaesthetist and surgeon were concerned the patient may develop a cement implantation reaction and required a quick surgery to reduce the risk of mortality.

3. What is the name of this implant?

This uncemented implant is the Austin-Moore. It is now rarely used and either more modern uncemented implants or a cemented implant would be used.

CASE 55: SLIPPED UPPER FEMORAL EPIPHYSIS

1. What are the risk factors for a patient developing an SUFE?

Risk factors include obesity and hypothyroidism.

2. What percentage of patients go on to develop a contralateral SUFE?

Approximately 25% of SUFE patients develop a contralateral SUFE. For this reason, prophylactic pinning is indicated in higher risk patients.

3. What are the key clinical features of an SUFE?

SUFEs can present as acute injury or more chronically and thus can present to a primary care physician or to the ED. Clinical features include shortening of the affected limb, external rotation of the limb and knee pain. In children presenting with knee pain, always think hip.

CASE 56: EWING'S SARCOMA

1. How common are primary malignant bone tumours in children?

Primary malignant bone tumours are exceedingly rare. Osteosarcoma is the most common malignant primary bone tumour in children and there are approximately 30 new cases of this per year in the UK.

2. **What are the red flag clinical features for a possible bone tumour?**

The red flag symptoms including night pain, progressive swelling/a new mass, disproportionate pain to the presenting complaint, loss of appetite, night sweats and unintended weight loss. While rare, the impact of a delayed diagnosis can be catastrophic and therefore it is always best to be cautious and refer/seek senior input if concerned.

3. **How is the treatment plan for a primary bone tumour decided?**

Every tumour will have to have a unique treatment plan based on its size, stage, location and histopathology and on the age of the patient. Therefore an MDT approach is required for managing these cases and surgery is one small but important part of that.

CASE 57: METASTATIC BONE DISEASE

1. **What cancers commonly metastasize to bone?**

The most common five cancers to metastasize to bone are breast, renal, lung, prostate and thyroid. Multiple myeloma may present with bone lesions. Increasingly, patients are presenting with metastatic disease from other cancers such as bowel cancer as the treatment improves and patients live longer.

2. **What radiological features of a bone lesion suggest cancer?**

Lesions which are suspicious for cancer are ill defined with a wide zone of transition, cortical erosion, surrounding soft tissue mass, periosteal reaction and/or an associated fracture.

3. **What factors need considered if planning surgical excision of a solitary bone metastasis?**

Some metastatic disease is now potentially curable. Solitary metastases can be excised as a part of wider course of treatment. An MDT is required to make the decision, but it is important to consider the location of the metastasis, whether it is surgically possible to reconstruct the skeleton after excision, for example, with a proximal femoral replacement and whether the tumour has an extensive blood supply. Sometimes an interventional radiologist is required to embolize the tumour before surgery to prevent haemorrhage.

CASE 58: NECK OF FEMUR FRACTURE/PAGET'S DISEASE

1. **What is Paget disease?**

Paget's disease is a disorder of bone turnover where there is excessive bone resorption and then abnormal new bone formation.

2. **What blood tests are required in assessing a patient with possible Paget disease?**

A high alkaline phosphatase with normal calcium levels, together with clinical and radiological changes, is highly suggestive of Paget disease. Clinical features include progressive bone deformity, bone pain, fractures and arthritis. A bone screen is required, and malignant conditions should be excluded.

3. **What is the treatment of Paget disease?**

Much of the treatment is supportive with the use of physiotherapy and analgesia. Bisphosphonates are the first-line treatment when patients are symptomatic. Surgery is only required if there is an associated fracture. Patients can develop high-output heart failure and therefore need to be investigated and treated for this as well.

CASE 59: ACETABULAR FRACTURE

1. **What other injuries should be considered when a patient presents with an acetabular fracture?**

These are high-energy injury fractures. There is a high risk the patient has any number of other injuries, some of which could be more urgent and life threatening. Therefore any patient who has an acetabular fracture (unless pathological) should have an ATLS ABCDE assessment.

2. **What is the treatment of choice for a displaced acetabular fracture?**

Displaced acetabular fractures generally require surgical fixation, especially in younger patients who have had a major trauma. However, the decision making is complex, and some fractures can be treated nonoperatively.

3. **What long-term issue may a patient develop following an acetabular fracture?**

Secondary arthritis is very common after an acetabular fracture. There is therefore an increasing interest in fixation of acetabular fractures with a hip replacement performed at the same time.

CASE 60: COMPLEX PELVIC FRACTURES

1. **What is the role of the pelvic binder in a trauma patient?**

Pelvic binders are potentially lifesaving tools in the trauma setting. Placed around the pelvis at the level of the greater trochanters, the binders are tightened to reduce and stabilize pelvic fractures. This can slow or stop major haemorrhage and therefore save lives. Once major haemorrhage has been excluded, and in discussion with the trauma team, the binder can be removed.

2. **What is Perthes disease?**

Perthes disease is a paediatric hip condition where there is avascular necrosis of the femoral head followed by a period of remodelling. It presents between the ages of 4 and 8 years and treatment is mainly supportive. The aim of treatment is to allow the condition to progress through these phases while maintaining a congruent hip joint with a spherical femoral head. Surgery is rarely required.

3. **What long-term issues could this patient develop because of their left hip?**

The femoral head is not spherical and therefore the hip is at risk of developing arthritis when the patient is older. A hip replacement would then be required, often at a younger age than is normal for hip arthritis.

CASE 61: AVASCULAR NECROSIS OF THE FEMORAL HEAD

1. **What are the causes of avascular necrosis?**

The most common cause idiopathic or unexplained. Other causes include steroid use, alcoholism, sickle cell disease, trauma, autoimmune conditions, radiotherapy and osteoarthritis.

2. **When performing a hip replacement, what surgical factors need to be considered specific to this patient?**
Patients who have been on steroids long term are at risk of poor wound healing and surgical site infection. Steroids can also cause a secondary osteoporosis, which may influence the surgical implant options.

3. **What condition could the patient develop after surgery if their steroid doses are not managed properly?**
Patients who have been on steroids for a long time are at risk of developing an Addisonian crisis because of the increased physiological stress of surgery. A temporary increase in steroid dosing around the time of surgery may be required to prevent this serious and potentially life-threatening condition from developing.

CASE 62: SUPERIOR AND INFERIOR PUBIC RAMI FRACTURES

1. **If there was a concern that the superior pubic ramus fracture extended into the acetabulum, what further imaging could be requested?**
A CT scan of the pelvis would give more information around the exact location of the fracture but is not required for this fracture.

2. **What anatomical structures pass through the obturator foramen?**
The obturator artery, vein and nerve pass through a gap in the obturator membrane called the *obturator canal*.

3. **What group of muscles originate for the ischial tuberosity?**
The hamstring muscles (semitendinosus, semimembranosus and biceps femoris) originate from the ischial tuberosity.

CASE 63: SUBTROCHANTERIC FRACTURE ASSOCIATED WITH LYTIC LESION

1. **What is the most likely cause of this fracture?**
A pathological fracture of this nature most likely represents a new diagnosis of metastatic disease and therefore a primary malignancy should be looked for.

2. **What are the advantages of early surgical fixation?**
Early fixation will provide pain relief, allow early mobilization and make nursing care easier. This will reduce the risks associated with a prolonged time in bed such as venous thrombotic events, chest infections and pressure sores.

3. **During intramedullary nailing, the patient develops sudden and severe hypoxia and hypotension. What is a particularly concerning cause?**
Fat embolism is a rare but life-threatening complication that can occur during intramedullary nailing. It is more common in prophylactic nailing where there is a bone lesion about to fracture. Fat from the marrow enters the blood stream and embolizing to the lungs causing hypoxia or to the brain causing reduced levels of consciousness. Treatment is supportive.

CASE 64: FEMORAL BONE LESION

1. **What are the four quadriceps muscles and what is their function?**
Rectus femoris, vastus lateralis, vastus intermedius and vastus medialis. The main role of the quadriceps is to extend the knee. Rectus femoris has attachments proximal to the hip and so flexes the hip as well.

2. **What structures are in Hunter's canal?**
Hunter's canal is a canal on the medial side of the knee bounded by sartorius, vastus medialis and adductor longus. It contains the femoral artery, femoral vein and saphenous nerve. Proximal to the knee, the saphenous nerve remains anterior and medial while the femoral artery and vein pass behind the knee to become the popliteal artery and vein.

3. **What radiological features suggest this bony lesion is malignant?**
There is a soft tissue mass, periosteal reaction, cortical destruction and a wide zone of transition.

CASE 65: MIDSHAFT FRACTURE OF FEMUR

1. **What are the benefits of applying traction to this limb following the injury?**
Traction prevents blood loss, fat embolism, provides pain relief and partially reduces the fracture before surgery.

2. **What device, invented in World War I, saved countless lives using traction?**
The Thomas Splint was invented in World War I and provided a mobile way of applying traction to a limb. It is estimated that the splint reduced the mortality rate following open femoral fractures from 80% to 20%.

3. **What features in the history suggest the patient should be investigated for underlying malignancy?**
Femoral shaft fractures are most commonly associated with high energy injuries. Therefore it is unusual to see this fracture following a fall from standing height. It may be that their age and diabetes point to osteoporosis, but it is best to investigate thoroughly and not miss a cancer diagnosis.

CASE 66: SCHATZKER TYPE 2 TIBIAL PLATEAU FRACTURE

1. **What are the four main ligaments of the knee?**
The four main ligaments are the medial collateral ligament, the lateral collateral ligament, the anterior cruciate ligament and the posterior cruciate ligament.

2. **What are the functions of these ligaments?**
The medial collateral ligament stabilizes the medial aspect of the knee providing resistance to valgus forces. The lateral collateral ligament stabilizes the lateral aspect of the knee providing resistance to varus forces. The anterior cruciate ligament stabilizes the knee again rotational forces and prevents anterior translation of the tibia in relation to the femur. The posterior cruciate ligament stabilizes the knee and prevents posterior translation of the tibia in relation to the femur.

3. **What serious and painful tibial condition may develop as a result of this injury?**
Tibial plateau fractures are often a result of high-energy trauma. There can be associated with significant soft tissue trauma, leading to swelling, bruising and rarely compartment syndrome.

CASE 67: TIBIA AND FIBULA SHAFT FRACTURES

1. **What is the function of the fibula?**
The fibula bears very little weight, and its main roles are in providing stability at the ankle and providing the origin for several muscles.

2. **What is the surgical treatment of choice for this patient?**

This fracture is best treated with an intramedullary nail. Because of the proximity to the ankle joint, it would be prudent to obtain a CT scan preoperatively as there is often a fracture line extending towards the ankle.

3. **The patient develops compartment syndrome. What treatment should they have?**

The treatment for acute compartment syndrome is surgery. The fascial compartments need to be opened up the length of the leg to adequately release the pressure and prevent muscle and nerve damage.

CASE 68: SCHATZKER TYPE 2 TIBIAL PLATEAU FRACTURE

1. **Why do tibial plateau fractures have a lipohaemarthrosis on X-ray?**

A lipohaemarthrosis is where both blood and fat cause an effusion. The presence of this on X-ray indicates a fracture even if one is not visible. The blood and fat come from within the bone and communicate with the joint.

2. **What are the potential complications that may occur from this fracture?**

Initially, there is a risk of compartment syndrome and soft tissue damage from the fracture. This is more common in higher energy tibial plateau fractures. There is a risk of nonunion or malunion. Malunion may lead to development of a valgus deformity and secondary arthritis.

3. **How might this fracture be fixed if surgery was considered?**

Intraarticular fractures require an anatomical reduction with a fixation that is rigid enough to hold the fracture reduced while allowing early mobilization. Implants now come anatomically precontoured with the option for fixation with screws that lock into the plate. Before applying the plate, the fracture must first be reduced and temporarily held with K wires.

CASE 69: SCHATZKER TYPE 1 TIBIAL PLATEAU FRACTURE

1. **When should surgery be considered for this fracture?**

If there is any significant displacement, then this fracture should be fixed to restore the articular surface, reduce the risk of nonunion and reduce the risk of future arthritis.

2. **How could this fracture be managed conservatively?**

They will require a hinged knee brace to limit but slowly increase range of motion and a period mobilizing non-weight bearing.

3. **What other considerations are required in managing this fracture conservatively?**

If the patient is mobilizing non-weight bearing, they are at an increased risk of a thrombotic event and thus should be provided with thromboprophylaxis. They will need to be taught how to use a brace and will require regular clinic follow-up to ensure fracture healing and that the position is maintained.

CASE 70: PATHOLOGICAL TIBIAL FRACTURE WITH ASSOCIATED BONE LESION

1. **What are the common benign bone tumours?**

The common benign bone tumours are simple bone cysts, enchondromas, aneurysmal bone cysts, giant cell tumours and fibrous cortical defects.

2. **What is the relevance of the location of the lesion in this case?**

Metastatic disease is very rare in the tibia. Any new bone tumour in the tibia is highly suspicious of a primary bone cancer such as osteosarcoma.

3. **What are the surgical treatment options for this lesion?**

The tumour and associated fracture need excision. As this is well below the knee, and the reconstruction options for the tibia are limited, this patient would likely undergo a below-knee amputation. This would need MDT discussion and a formal diagnosis before any surgery.

CASE 71: TIBIA AND FIBULA SPIRAL FRACTURES

1. **What are the immediate life-threatening complications of trauma that an ABCDE assessments looks to identify or exclude?**

A, look for airway obstruction; B, look for pneumothoraces (tension, simple or open), haemothoraces, a flail chest with pulmonary contusion, and cardiac tamponade; C, particularly looking for haemorrhage, which could be from the chest, abdomen (including retroperitoneal space), pelvis, long bones or externally (on the floor); D, look for brain injury; E, the exposure component is important to make sure a thorough and complete examination has been completed (although it is unlikely to identify a life-threatening injury that has not already been picked up).

2. **What are the clinical examination findings that suggest compartment syndrome?**

Compartment syndrome presents with severe unremitting pain that is not controlled by strong analgesia and is exacerbated by passive flexion or extension of the toes or fingers. The compartment will feel hard like wood. The other signs of neurovascular compromise late but patients may present with altered sensation. It is unusual for there to be no pulse.

3. **Which other surgical specialty may need to be involved after the fasciotomies?**

Fasciotomy wounds need to be left open and dressed appropriately while swelling resolves. Over time, closure of the wound can be attempted but often plastic surgery is required to apply skin grafts to the wounds. These wounds leave a lot of scarring, but the alternative is severe muscle and nerve damage with loss of function in the limb if compartment syndrome is missed.

CASE 72: COMMINUTED PATELLA FRACTURE

1. **What is the function of the patella?**

The patella is a sesamoid bone within the extensor/quadriceps mechanism. The patella increases the moment arm for the quadriceps, which improves the function of the muscle.

2. **What examination finding suggests fracture of the patella or extensor mechanism disruption?**

If the patella is fractured or if there is a tear of the quadriceps or patella tendon, the patient is unable to perform a straight leg raise.

3. **What late complication can occur because of this fracture and how might it present?**

This is an intraarticular fracture and so the patient is at risk of developing secondary arthritis. This would present with pain at the front of the knee. Pain would be worse where forces through the patella are increased through activities such as walking up and down stairs.

CASE 73: ANTERIOR KNEE DISLOCATION WITH ASSOCIATED TIBIAL AVULSION FRACTURE

1. **For a knee to dislocate, which two of the four main ligaments must have ruptured?**

For the tibiofemoral joint to dislocate the anterior and posterior cruciate ligament must both rupture. However, it is common for three if not all four ligaments to rupture in the same injury.

2. **Presuming there is a vascular injury, while the vascular surgeons restore blood supply, what may need to be applied to the limb to maintain a reduced and stable knee?**

An external fixator may be required temporarily to keep the knee stable while the limb is reperfused. Definitive reconstructive surgery should be performed at a later date.

3. **What prophylactic operation should also be performed at the time of reperfusion of the limb?**

When a limb has had a period of ischaemia and is reperfused, significant swelling can occur leading to compartment syndrome. Therefore fasciotomies should be considered to prevent this from occurring.

CASE 74: OSTEOCHONDROMATA

1. **What is an exostosis?**

An exostosis is an abnormal growth of cartilage and bone and is sometimes called an *osteochondroma*. There arise from the growth plate and extend away from the joint. The cortex of the lesion is in continuity with the cortex of normal bone. Most are asymptomatic and so the true prevalence is unknown.

2. **What is the risk of malignant transmission in multiple hereditary exostoses (MHE)?**

MHE is an autosomal dominant inherited condition associated with the *EXT-1*, *EXT-2* and *EXT-3* genes. Unlike solitary exostoses where malignant transformation to a chondrosarcoma is extremely rare, the risk of malignant transmission is 5% in MHE.

3. **What is the surgical management of a simple solitary exostosis?**

Most exostoses are asymptomatic and can be left alone. Some do cause localized tenderness depending on their location. They can present with nerve pain if they are close to a nerve, for example, the fibular head and common peroneal nerve. Excision is usually curative, but the tumour can recur.

CASE 75: OSTEOCHONDRAL DEFECT WITH ASSOCIATED LOOSE BODY

1. **What is the blood supply to articular cartilage?**

There is no blood supply to the cartilage. It is avascular and aneural. Therefore it has no potential for healing.

2. **Why is fixation of the osteochondral fragment unlikely to be successful?**

The patient is 4 months post injury. The osteochondral fragment will have changed shape and been damaged over time. Scar tissue will have formed in its place. Some surgeons would still advocate trying as its best to try and repair osteochondral defects but the chance for successful healing is much lower.

3. **What is microfracture and how does it work?**

Microfracture is a treatment for articular cartilage defects. First the margins of the defect are stabilized. Next the bone surface is exposed. A microfracture pick is used to make multiple holes in the bone with the aim of stimulating bleeding and healing with the formation of a fibrocartilage.

CASE 76: SEGOND TIBIAL PLATEAU FRACTURE

1. **What shock absorbing cartilage in the knee is commonly injured in ACL injuries?**

The menisci of the knee are sometimes referred to as the *shock absorbing* or *footballers' cartilage of the knee*. When torn, the meniscus is unable to transmit forces through the knee effectively. The meniscus also provides stability to the knee. It is important to assess for and treat meniscal tears as part of ACL injury management with the goal of repairing a torn meniscus where possible.

2. **What are the clinical examination tests that assess the ACL?**

Three tests for ACL deficiency are commonly used. For the anterior drawer test, the knee is positioned at 90 degrees. The examiner sits on the patient's foot and pulls the tibia forward in relation to femur. Lachman's test is similar to the anterior draw but at 30 degrees of flexion. Marked translation of the tibia in relation to the femur is elicited in a positive test. The Pivot shift test tests for rotational instability. The leg is extended, the foot internally rotated and a valgus force is applied to the knee. The knee is then flexed, and a visible and sometimes audible clunk can be seen or heard.

3. **What is the treatment of choice for a young athlete with an ACL rupture?**

Young athletic patients with an ACL rupture who want to return to sports are best treated with early injury recognition, prehabilitation and then ACL reconstruction. This is followed by extensive rehabilitation.

CASE 77: HYPERTROPHIC OSTEOARTHROPATHY

1. **What is the main ligament that stabilizes the medial side of the ankle?**

The deltoid ligament. This ligament is made up of superficial and deep layers.

2. **What are the main ligaments that stabilize the syndesmosis?**

The syndesmosis is stabilized by the anterior inferior tibiofibular ligament, the interosseous ligament, the posterior inferior tibiofibular ligament and transverse tibiofibular ligament.

3. **What ligament is commonly injured in an ankle sprain?**

Ankle sprains commonly affect the lateral side. The lateral ligaments are the anterior talofibular ligament, calcaneofibular ligament and posterior talofibular ligament.

CASE 78: DISTAL TIBIA AND FIBULA FRACTURES

1. **What are the advantages of treating this fracture nonoperatively?**

Nonoperative treatment avoids the risk of an anaesthetic and there is no risk of a surgical complication such as infection. There is no risk of damaging adjacent structures while placing the plate and there is no need to have to consider future plate removal.

2. **What are the disadvantages of treating this fracture nonoperatively?**

Maintaining the fracture in an adequate position can be more difficult in plaster. The patient will require multiple visits to the fracture clinic for X-rays to ensure the position is maintained. The patient will not be able to put weight through the limb, which could lead to an extended stay in hospital or rehabilitation unit. If the fracture does not heal in a good position, it could affect function long term.

3. **An anterior approach to the ankle is made to fix the fracture. What neurovascular structures may be encountered and need protecting?**

The neurovascular structures, which need protecting during an anterior approach to the ankle are the anterior tibial artery, the deep peroneal nerve and more laterally and superficially the superficial peroneal nerve.

CASE 79: WEBER A ANKLE FRACTURE

1. **What is the Weber classification for ankle fractures?**

The Weber classification describes the location of the fibula fracture in relation to the syndesmosis. This can be helpful in predicting the management of the fracture.

2. **What is the mechanism of injury for Weber A ankle fractures?**

Weber A fractures are below the syndesmosis and represent an avulsion of the distal fibular. It is the same mechanisms as a severe ankle sprain but instead of the ligaments rupturing, the bone fractures.

3. **What is the treatment of choice for Weber A fractures?**

Weber A fractures can be treated nonoperatively. The ankle joint is stable and can bear weight. The fractures almost always go on to unite. A walking boot can be provided for pain relief with follow-up at 6 weeks to ensure the fracture has healed.

CASE 80: WEBER B ANKLE FRACTURE

1. **What is the definition of a Weber B fracture?**

A Weber B fracture is an ankle fracture where the fibular is fractured at the level of the syndesmosis. While some Weber B fractures do need surgery others do not, so it is important to assess other radiological features like the medial clear space.

2. **What nerve is at risk during the surgical approach to the fibular?**

A lateral approach is commonly used. The superficial peroneal nerve is close to the approach and can inadvertently be cut during surgery. This would lead to a numb patch on the dorsum of the foot.

3. **What ligament attaches at the level of this fracture between the tibia and fibula anteriorly?**

The anterior inferior tibiofibular ligament. This is one of four ligaments, which make up the syndesmosis. This is the name given the ligamentous complex that stabilizes the distal tibiofibular joint.

CASE 81: WEBER C ANKLE FRACTURE

1. **What is the definition of a Weber C ankle fracture?**

A Weber C fracture is one above the level of the syndesmosis. These are almost always associated with instability in the ankle joint because of rupture of the syndesmosis and require surgical fixation.

2. **What fixation needs to be performed along with fixation of the fibular fracture?**

Syndesmosis fixation is required along with fixation of the fibular. If the medial malleolus is fractured, this requires fixation also. The syndesmosis is normally fixed with either a screw or a tightrope suture through the fibular and tibia.

3. **How would this fixation impact on rehab?**

This ligamentous component of the injury normally requires more time before starting rehabilitation. This is particularly the case with screw fixation where early mobilization may lead to the screw backing out, breaking or becoming loose.

CASE 82: WEBER B ANKLE FRACTURE

1. **What other ligaments make up the syndesmosis?**

The main ligaments are the anterior inferior tibiofibular ligament, interosseous ligament and posterior inferior distal tibiofibular ligament.

2. **What is the importance of the impaction injury to the anterior tibia?**

The impaction is quite small, and it would be difficult to reduce this and hold it surgically with a plate or screws. This represents the damage to the ankle joint that occurs at the time of injury. This is in part why despite best efforts, some patients will go on to develop arthritis in the ankle.

3. **Why does this fracture require surgical fixation?**

The ankle joint is not congruent as demonstrated by the widened medial clear space. Greater than 2-mm incongruence is associated with abnormal loads through the joint, which leads to loss of function and secondary arthritis. An anatomical reduction should be the aim for all ankle fractures.

CASE 83: MAISONNEUVE ANKLE FRACTURE

1. **What clinical test can be used to test for syndesmosis disruption?**

   The squeeze test involves squeezing the tibia and fibular together. Pain felt at the ankle joint suggests a syndesmosis disruption.

2. **Does the fibular need fixation in this patient?**

   The fibular does not require fixation. More proximal fibular fracture as seen in the Masionneuve injury can be left alone and attention turned towards reducing the syndesmosis, reducing the medial clear space and restoring articular congruence.

3. **What will the long-term effects be of not repairing the syndesmosis?**

   Malreduction and malunion of the syndesmosis leads to pain, loss of function and secondary arthritis.

CASE 84: TRIMALLEOLAR ANKLE FRACTURE WITH DISLOCATION OF THE TIBIOTALAR JOINT

1. **On which side of the ankle is it more likely that the fracture will become open, medial or lateral?**

   Ankle fractures most commonly displace into a valgus position with the medial malleoulus tenting the skin and it is at this site that the fracture is most likely to puncture the skin and become a compound fracture. This is important as this is the site to examine most carefully to ensure a small puncture wound is not missed.

2. **In this case, the patient has significant swelling. What is the risk of performing surgery at this stage?**

   The skin is prone to not healing around the ankle. If the skin is already damaged and swollen from a significant ankle fracture and dislocation, then while it may be possible to reduce the bones back into place the wound may not heal or it may become infected. This can be very difficult to treat.

3. **What alternative surgical option is available if definitive fixation cannot be performed?**

   If the soft tissue swelling is too severe and the fracture too unstable for a plaster cast, then an external fixator can be used temporarily to allow swelling to settle before fixation. This process normally takes a week to 10 days of rest, ice and elevation on the ward.

CASE 85: MEDIAL MALLEOLUS FRACTURE

1. **What complication are medial malleolus fractures prone to?**

   Medial malleoli fractures have a high rate of nonunion. Even if minimally displaced, consideration is given to fixation to prevent this from happening.

2. **What structure originates from the medial malleolus and stabilizes the ankle on the medial side?**

   The Deltoid ligament.

3. **What is the cause for this complication?**

   There are a number of reasons for nonunion, but specifically in medial malleoli fractures what happens is that as the fracture occurs, periosteum and the deltoid ligament come away at the fracture and lodge within the fracture line blocking bony healing. At the time of surgery, it is therefore important to remove this soft tissue from the fracture.

CASE 86: FRACTURE AT BASE OF FIFTH METATARSAL

1. **What injuries are associated with base of 5th metatarsal fractures?**

   Fifth metatarsal injuries are often associated with lateral ankle ligament laxity or injury. Often it can be difficult to differentiate if the pain is from the fibular or the 5th metatarsal.

2. **What is the eponymous name given to base of 5th metatarsal fractures?**

   Fifth metatarsal fractures are sometimes called *Jones fractures*. The eponym refers to a distinct anatomical region at the base of the 5th metatarsal where there is a poorer blood supply and a higher rate of nonunion.

3. **What tendon inserts into the base of the 5th metatarsal?**

   The peroneus brevis tenson inserts into the base of the 5th metatarsal. Peroneus brevis provides dynamic stability to the lateral aspect of the ankle hence why this fracture has a similar mechanism of injury as an ankle sprain.

CASE 87: PEDUNCULATED BONE LESION

1. **Where might this patient experience numbness if the lesion was compressing a nerve?**

   The deep peroneal nerve will be close to this lesion and if compressed, then the patient would experience numbness in the first web space of the foot.

2. **What tendons pass anterior to the ankle?**

   The muscles of the anterior compartment of the leg are tibialis anterior, extensor hallucis longus and extensor digitorum longus.

3. **What are the functions of these tendons?**

   Tibialis anterior is responsible for ankle dorsiflexion, extensor hallucis longus for big toe extension and extensor digitorum longus lesser toe extension.

CASE 88: NORMAL PAEDIATRIC FOOT

1. **What is an apophysis?**

   An apophysis is a secondary bone ossification centre that forms a protuberance on a bone, and often has tendon attachments. Another example is the greater trochanter of the femur.

2. **What is the nerve supply to peroneus brevis?**

   The superficial peroneal nerve innervates the muscles of the lateral compartment of the leg and this includes peroneus brevis.

3. **What is the other peroneal muscle and what is its function?**

   The other peroneal muscle in the lateral compartment of the leg is peroneus longus. This muscle attaches to the base of the 1st metatarsal. When contracted the muscle creates flexion and eversion of the foot.

CASE 89: INTRAARTICULAR CALCANEAL FRACTURE

1. **When a person falls from a significant height what major orthopaedic injuries commonly occur?**

   Following a fall from a significant height in theory any injury is possible, but the common injuries encountered include calcaneal fractures, comminuted intraarticular distal tibial fractures (pilon fractures), vertical shear pelvic fractures and spinal fractures.

2. What is the mechanism for the secondary fracture in this case?

This is an avulsion fracture. They occur at the insertion of a tendon or ligament where the tendon or ligament has been pulled off with a piece of bone.

3. What tendon inserts into the calcaneum at the site of this fracture?

The Achilles tendon has a broad insertion on the posterior aspect of the calcaneum.

CASE 90: METATARSAL BASE FRACTURES WITH ASSOCIATED LISFRANC INJURY

1. What is Lisfranc's ligament?

The Lisfranc ligament attaches the base of the 2nd metatarsal bone to the medial cuneiform.

2. Why is the Lisfranc ligament important?

The midfoot bones function as a roman arch. Without the Lisfranc ligament, the midfoot becomes unstable causing subluxations or dislocations of the tarsometatarsal joints (depending on severity of the injury). This leads to pain, dysfunction and secondary arthritis.

3. What is the classical clinical feature of a Lisfranc injury?

While more severe injuries present with pain, significant swelling and are readily diagnosed, less severe but still very significant injuries can be missed. Plantar ecchymosis is pathognomonic for a Lisfranc injury. Therefore it is important to examine the whole foot following an injury.

CASE 91: FRACTURE OF THE PROXIMAL PHALANX

1. What is the treatment of choice for the majority of lesser toe fractures?

Nearly all toe fractures can be treated with some form of splinting. This can be buddy strapping or a short walking boot. The only indication for surgery would be an open fracture.

2. What is a hammer toe deformity?

In a hammer toe deformity, there is flexion of the proximal interphalangeal joint with extension of the metatarsophalangeal joint.

3. What is a mallet toe deformity?

In a mallet toe deformity, there is flexion of the distal interphalangeal joint.

CASE 92: MEDIAL SUB-TALAR DISLOCATION

1. What structures are on the medial side of the ankle posterior to the medial malleolus?

Behind the medial malleolus, within the tarsal tunnel, are tibialis posterior, flexor digitorum longus, posterior tibial artery and vein, the tibial nerve and flexor hallucis longus. Some people use the mnemonic 'Tom, Dick, and A Very Nervous Harry' to remember the order.

2. What four bones does the talus articulate with?

The talus articulates with the distal tibia, the fibula, the calcaneum and the navicular. Each joint function is complex but crucial for load transmission and a normal gait.

3. Which muscles or tendons attach to the talus?

No muscles or tendons attach to the talus. This is partly why it is possible for the talus to dislocate completely from all its articulations in what is called a *total talar extrusion*. It also means the talus receives no blood supply through these insertions.

CASE 93: INTRAOSSEOUS LIPOMA

1. What radiological features suggest this is a benign lesion?

The lesion is a narrow zone of transition. There is no cortical destruction. There is no periosteal reaction and there is no associated soft tissue mass.

2. What is the differential diagnosis for this lesion?

An intraosseous lipoma is the most likely diagnosis because of the appearances but also because they are most common in the calcaneum. Differentials would include other benign bone cysts such as a simple bone cyst.

3. If symptomatic, how might it be treated?

Most are asymptomatic and can be left. However, if the patient does have symptoms, the lesion can be treated with curettage and bone grafting.

CASE 94: METATARSAL STRESS FRACTURE

1. What conditions or activities are associated with stress fractures?

Repetitive trauma from long distance running or walking (the fracture is sometimes called a *Marcher's fracture*), osteopaenia/osteoporosis from a poor diet or metabolic disorder, or an associated deformity of the foot are all associated with stress fractures.

2. What is the treatment of choice for most metatarsal fractures?

Unless there are multiple metatarsal fractures or a fracture that is widely displaced then metatarsal fractures can be treated nonoperatively. A short period of immobilization in a walking boot with weight bearing as pain allows is advised. Most patients do not require follow-up as the fracture normally heals.

3. What may be required if a patient has had multiple stress fractures?

If a patient is having recurrent metatarsal stress fractures, then close attention should be paid to their diet or the shape of their foot. Athletes sometimes can present with a triad of anorexia, amenorrhoea and stress fractures and this requires MDT care. If the patient has a high arched (cavovarus) foot, then surgical correction of the foot deformity may be required.

CASE 95: AVULSION FRACTURE AT THE METATARSAL BASE

1. What two joints are there at the base of the 5th metatarsal?

There is the cubometatarsal joint and the 4th/5th intermetatarsal joint.

2. What is the plantar fascia?

The plantar fascia is a thick band of tissue that runs from the calcaneum to the toes. On the calcaneum, its main attachment is to the calcaneal tuberosity, which is on the medial plantar aspect.

3. What is the function of the plantar fascia?

The fascia supports the arches of the foot when walking and can become inflamed causing a plantar fasciitis. Pain is felt at its origin on the calcaneum and pinpoint tenderness at the calcaneal tuberosity is pathognomonic of plantar fasciitis.

CASE 96: CHARCOT FOOT

1. What are the causes of a Charcot joint?

This condition occurs because of a neuropathy that affects the ability to protect the foot/ankle from multiple microtraumas. This leads to destruction of the foot and ankle joints, creating a deformity and loss of function in the foot.

Any condition that causes a neuropathy (alcoholism, myelomeningocele) can cause this, but diabetes is the most common cause.

2. What is the aim of treating this condition in a total contact casting?

The condition goes through stages of destruction and then healing. Total contact casting aims to maintain the foot in a shoeable shape so that once resolved, the patient can still walk and wear shoes while minimizing the risk of developing ulcers.

3. When may surgery be required in these patients?

If casting does not work, then surgery may be required to remove bony spurs or correct a deformity. The decision making for the surgery is complex and there will be variation in the deformity needing treated. Occasionally, if all else fails amputation may be considered.

CASE 97: FREIBERG'S DISEASE OF THE METATARSAL

1. What is Freiberg's disease?

Freiberg's disease is an osteochondrosis characterized by infarction and deformity of the 2nd and occasionally, 3rd metatarsal heads.

2. What other osteochondroses/apophysitis can occur in the foot?

Kohler's disease is a condition where there is avascular necrosis of the navicular. Sever's disease is a traction apophysitis of the calcaneum.

3. What is the mainstay of treatment for these conditions and why?

These conditions can be treated with a period of rest with or without splinting using a short walking boot or a cast. The vast majority resolve with time. Surgery is rarely required although it is occasionally used in Freiberg's disease to try and help maintain the shape of the 2nd metatarsal head.

CASE 98: GOUT

1. What is gout?

Gout is an inflammatory arthritis where there is intraarticular urate crystal deposition. This leads to recurrent acute attacks of pain and swelling at the affected joint. Over time, this leads to joint destruction and secondary arthritis formation.

2. Which joints are commonly affected?

The small joints of the hand and foot with the 1st metatarsal phalangeal joint being most common. This is unlike pseudogout where the crystals are calcium pyrophosphate. This affects larger joints including most commonly the knee.

3. What is the treatment of gout?

Acute gout flares should be treated with antiinflammatories such as indomethacin or colchicine. Chronic gout treatment includes allopurinol with the aim of preventing further acute flares. Occasionally, steroids are used in severe cases.

CASE 99: OSTEOMYELITIS

1. Why does a diabetic patient develop nonhealing ulcers?

Diabetes causes both macrovascular and microvascular disease. This means that blood flow to tissues is impaired on both a macrovascular and microvascular level and healing is delayed or not possible. This together with the loss of protective sensation increases the risk of developing an ulcer that does not heal.

2. What is the name given to an amputation through the ankle joint?

This is called a *Syme's amputation*. Amputations at various levels of the foot and leg are well described and each have their advantages and disadvantages.

3. How is the level of amputation decided?

The limb needs to be amputated at the best level possible to preserve function while ensuring that there is the potential for healing at the level amputated and no remaining infection in the tissues.

CASE 100: SALTER-HARRIS TYPE 3 PHALANX FRACTURE

1. What is the Salter-Harris classification of fractures around the growth plates?

The classification runs from 1 to 5: 1 is straight through the growth plate; 2 is a fracture line through the growth plate with a bony fragment away from the joint; 3 is a fracture line through the growth plate with a bony fragment towards the joint; 4 is a fracture line extending both into and away from the joint; 5 is a crush injury to the growth plate.

2. What important complication is associated with Salter-Harris fractures affecting the growth plate?

When there is a fracture line extending towards the joint or a crush to the growth plate (types 3–5), there is an increased risk of growth arrest.

3. What tendon inserts to the dorsum of the big toe distal phalanx?

Extensor hallucis longus inserts here and extends the big toe.

Case Index

Index

Note: Page numbers followed by *f* indicate figures.